Rehabilitation Interventions for the Institutionalized Elderly

Rehabilitation Interventions for the Institutionalized Elderly

Ellen D. Taira
Editor

The Haworth Press
New York • London

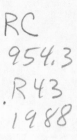

Rehabilitation Interventions for the Institutionalized Elderly has also been published as *Physical & Occupational Therapy in Geriatrics*, Volume 6, Number 2, 1988.

The Haworth Press, Inc., 12 West 32 Street, New York, NY 10001
EUROSPAN/Haworth, 3 Henrietta Street, London WC2E 8LU England

LIBRARY OF CONGRESS
Library of Congress Cataloging-in-Publication Data

Rehabilitation interventions for the institutionalized elderly / Ellen D. Taira, editor.
    p. cm.
    "Has also been published as Physical & occupational therapy in geriatrics, volume 6, number 2, 1988" — T.p. verso.
    Includes bibliographies and index.
    ISBN 0-86656-833-6
    1. Aged — Institutional care. 2. Aged — Rehabilitation. I. Taira, Ellen D.
    [DNLM: 1. Homes for the Aged. 2. Nursing Homes. 3. Rehabilitation — in old age. W1 PH683M v. 6 no. 2 / WT 30 R345] RC854.3.R43 1988
362.6'1 — dc 19
DNI M/DLC
for Library of Congress

88-18065
CIP

Rehabilitation Interventions for the Institutionalized Elderly

CONTENTS

ABOUT THE EDITOR

Ellen Dunleavy Taira, OTR, MPH, is affiliated with New York University Medical Center as Assistant Director of the Occupational Therapy Department at Goldwater Memorial Hospital, a 900 bed chronic-care facility in New York City. She has practiced as an occupational therapist specializing in gerontology for more than 20 years with expertise in many areas of long term care. Ms. Taira is the editor of *Physical & Occupational Therapy in Geriatrics*.

FROM THE EDITOR

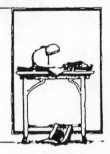

This is the first issue of *POTG* to focus exclusively on rehabilitation services for the institutionalized elderly. Although institutions are the traditional domain of physical and occupational therapists, there has been a strong move towards more community health services in the last decade. Few dispute the argument that services provided in the least restrictive environment are usually preferred by the older person and often represent the most humane approach. Nevertheless, the cost effectiveness issue remains unresolved. During a recent session at the 40th annual meeting of the Gerontological Society of America (1987), there were some very articulate spokespersons for the less academic and more pragmatic approach to the community versus institution issue. Clearly, the essential role of the nursing home in the long term care continuum will undoubtedly continue even as community services expand. This is particularly the case in an era of DRGs and the prudent use of costly acute care. Patients are being discharged "quicker and sicker" and many of them find their way to a Skilled Nursing Facility (SNF) for a continuation of their treatment in a less intensive and expensive setting.

There is an immediate need to enrich the quality of rehabilitation services offered to the institutionalized elderly. The role of rehabilitation specialists is growing rapidly with only the supply of therapists a limiting factor.

Current trends in geriatric rehabilitation has been the theme of *POTG* during the tenure of this editor. This issue contains an especially interesting selection of studies and ideas that would have been unlikely even a few years ago. The lead article on Rehabilitation Advocacy should start us all thinking about where we should be directing our energy in the next few years. There is little room for complacency if we are to carve out a place for geriatric rehabilitation in the next decade.

There follows three distinctly different but related studies on the response of elderly persons to therapeutic interventions. Howard investigated the older person's response to touch and found touch did positively affect their participation in an occupational therapy activity. Christopher studied patients' response to group psychotherapy and noted some small but observable gains in the direction of discharge planning. Most importantly for therapists was the increased involvement of the patient in decision making, something that can and should be incorporated into their daily treatment prior to discharge. Lastly, Lushbough and colleagues studied the response of psychogeriatric patients to verbal and activity interventions. Once again, unexpected gains related to discharge planning were noted.

Breines took a familiar treatment intervention in a nursing home setting, namely teaching wheelchair mobility, and presented a refreshing new look at the value of this activity to the older person from a sensorimotor perspective. Ryan's technological adaptation article also addresses mobility but for a cognitively intact person who has few opportunities for functional independence other than mobility. This is a subject of great interest to me and of tremendous significance in the field of gerontology where technology has been a mixed blessing to chronically ill persons.

Lastly, a new section, "Another Perspective," has been added to *POTG* to address the sometimes neglected personal concerns that older persons and therapists often think about but rarely put in print.

Your comments and personal reflections are welcome.

EDT

Rehabilitation Advocacy:
A New Role for Therapists
Working with the Elderly

Jeffrey L. Crabtree, OTR

Our society is experiencing a population growth that could soon rock its very foundation. According to the Bureau of the Census, the population aged 65 and over grew twice as fast as the rest of the American population between 1960 and 1980 and is projected to double between 1980 and 2020 (Schick, 1986). By 2020, Census estimates that there will be 51.4 million people 65 years or older and 7.1 million of those will be 85 years old or over (Schick, 1986). Where will they live and receive their health care? According to The Division of Health Care Studies, National Nursing Home Survey, about 20% of the 85 and older live in nursing homes (National Center for Health Statistics, 1985). At 1985 rates of mortality and nursing home use, we will need to build between 320 and 600 new 100-bed nursing homes each year for the next 15 years to keep up with the demand (Riche, 1985). This dramatic change in demographics will challenge our society on many levels. One of these is the health care system and especially the effective rehabilitation of the elderly.

NURSING HOMES: THE REHABILITATION INSTITUTION FOR THE ELDERLY

For many people, including those of us in the health care field, the nursing home is considered the last stop for the elderly, a place where old people go to die. Even to the extent this is partially true,

---

Jeffrey L. Crabtree, Northern Division Director, Therapy Management.

it need not be the only truth about nursing homes. The length of stay in acute hospitals from 1968 to 1983 has decreased from 8.5 to 6.9 days per patient (National Center for Health Care Statistics, 1985). There has been a 25% increase in the number of nursing home beds from 1969 to 1983 and a general decline in the number of acute care beds for the same period (National Center for Health Care Statistics, 1985). These trends, which represent a shift in utilization of acute hospital and nursing home care, may lead to a significant change in how society views nursing homes. The nursing home may become the "centerpiece" of the long-term health care system of the future (Levenson, 1987). Rehabilitation specialists have an exciting opportunity to facilitate that change in attitude about nursing homes.

In order to take a leadership role in this much needed change, therapists must broaden the traditional therapist-patient role to include becoming advocates of rehabilitation of the elderly. There are five areas for which strategies must be developed.

1. The elderly must be able to ask for and recognize quality rehabilitation.
2. Referral sources in the health care system must refer appropriately to quality rehabilitation programs.
3. Third party payors must be willing to pay for rehabilitation services.
4. Nursing home owners and administrators must see the value in providing quality rehabilitation services.
5. Rehabilitation specialists must ensure that rehabilitation services are effective.

THE ELDERLY AS ENLIGHTENED CONSUMERS

Recognition of the need for rehabilitation services for the elderly seems to be based more upon the awareness of health care professionals than upon the elderly's awareness of their own need for services (Johnson, 1987). The elderly need to understand what is available to them and what benefits they can expect from rehabilitation.

Therapists can do much to help these end users of rehabilitation appropriately identify and articulate their needs. We must help society and especially the elderly to learn what rehabilitation is, how to recognize quality rehabilitation and when to demand quality rehabilitation. Following are some examples of how to inform the elderly in your community about the value of rehabilitation.

Speak at Senior Centers

Most communities have at least one service organization for the elderly such as a senior center or a senior's church group. Contact these community agencies and centers. Volunteer to speak to their patrons on practical subjects like safety in the home, help to care givers, what to expect when a spouse has a stroke and similar topics. Ask the representative of the service organization what topics appear to be of the greatest interest. Invite other members of your health care community, such as your nursing home administrator or local pharmacist, to speak with you. When you present to these groups of elders offer them examples of good rehabilitation and of positive outcomes from nursing home admissions.

Utilize Elders in the Community

Look for older citizens in your community who are active and interested in helping others. These folks can be found in dance or social clubs, community colleges, church groups and in organizations such as the American Association of Retired Persons. A square dancing club, for example, might be willing to put on a demonstration of square dancing in your nursing home. In cooperation with the activities department, create a Western theme open house and invite family members, neighbors and local officials, such as City Council members. Use this opportunity to demonstrate the values of rehabilitation to the elderly. Make sure the guests get a tour of the nursing facility and an opportunity to meet the staff and residents.

Contact Retirement Centers

There is likely to be a retirement center near you. Contact the manager and offer to speak to the residents on various topics of interest. Explore the need for self-help groups such as a stroke support group, or an arthritis self-help group. When appropriate, offer to help establish such a group or offer to put these retirees in touch with local resource persons such as occupational, speech and physical therapists.

Utilize Local Nursing Homes

Through local nursing homes, offer annual free or low cost services to the elderly in the community. These could include general health screenings, blood pressure, vision and hearing screenings, or consumer seminars on rehabilitation and health issues. Community professionals will recognize the promotional value of these activities and appreciate the opportunity to provide the service. Such activities help to bring the well elderly and family members to the nursing home and provide them an opportunity to meet staff and residents. These wellness activities are also opportunities to demonstrate to the community that nursing homes can be dynamic institutions that foster health in the aging population.

Resources

Many local and national service organizations will provide you with free or reasonably priced literature on a variety of topics important to the elders in your community. Your local or national professional organization such as the American Occupational Therapy Association publishes brochures and other materials suitable for distribution to elder groups. Hand these out when speaking before groups and when hosting open houses and seminars.

HEALTH CARE PROVIDERS AS ENLIGHTENED REFERRAL SOURCES

While it is important that the elderly be able to recognize quality rehabilitation, we must not neglect the education of the physicians, discharge planners, nursing home administrators, third party payors and others who share the responsibility of improving access to rehabilitation. These players in the health care system should know enough about rehabilitation and its component parts to support the elderly consumer when he or she asks for rehabilitation services.

The techniques for educating providers are quite similar to those used in formal marketing and promotion. Contact your professional association to get ideas and materials that will help you inform health care providers about the value of rehabilitation to the elderly.

Presentations

Formal papers discussing the value of rehabilitation and the team approach to rehabilitation can be presented to a variety of groups such as the Arthritis Foundation, the American Society on Aging, The American Health Care Association, The National Institute of Aging, and many other local and national associations. Present informal talks to your local professional societies or special interest groups. Many of our own peers are unaware of the need for or value of rehabilitation of the elderly.

Share Your Experiences

Take every opportunity to share positive outcomes with your patient's family, attending physician and other referral sources. For example, invite family members to observe treatment. Send progress notes to the attending physician and thank him for the opportunity to treat his patient. Send copies of reports to the discharge planner who referred the patient. Use a brief cover letter that identifies the patient's new abilities or level of independence. Contact your local newspaper when significant rehabilitation events occur. Press releases to health editors in the print media can be useful. Prepare releases on topics such as the 100th birthday of a resident, open houses, consumer related seminars, health screenings and other activities that would be of interest to the public. Offer to discuss your professional view of rehabilitation at local long-term or acute care facility inservices. Use those occasions to praise individuals who have done a good job in helping to rehabilitate the elderly.

THIRD PARTY PAYORS
AS ENLIGHTENED CONSUMERS

Reviewers for private insurance companies and for Medicare intermediaries are critically important members of the health care system. They can be exposed to the value of rehabilitation and its component parts most effectively through meaningful and concise documentation of rehabilitation services. After all, they are reviewing records for their insurance company. They want to know that they are paying for valued services. When they read carefully written notes that indicate a clear treatment plan and well documented treatment activities that lead to a reasonable rehabilitation outcome, they will see the value of rehabilitation.

Call these reviewers when you have questions about coverage and when you can share your successes with them. Get to know these individuals by inviting them to your facility's open house and other functions. Often they will appreciate the opportunity to see where the services are provided and to meet with patients and staff.

NURSING HOME ADMINISTRATORS AS ENLIGHTENED PROVIDERS

Nursing home administrators need to recognize the practical value that participation in the Medicare program has for many of their residents. Medicare is the largest single health care insurer of the population 65 and older (President's Commission for the Study of Ethical Problems in Medicine and Biomedical and Behavioral Research, 1983). Despite this potential for reimbursement of rehabilitation services, many nursing home administrators choose not to participate in the Medicare system. The administrator's reasons for not participating may be that the facility does not meet structural requirements, that too much paperwork is involved, that the nursing staff would object or that Medicare does not pay adequately. Some reasons are quite valid, but the rehabilitation practitioner should question the nursing home administrator's preconceptions about Medicare and help him get the information he needs to make informed decisions.

Utilize your national or state association to develop persuasive information to present to your nursing home administrator to demonstrate the clinical advantages of participating in the Medicare program. Contact your nearest Regional Office of the Health Care Financing Administration. This is the federal agency that administers the Medicare program. Identify an individual who would be willing to discuss participation in the program with your administrator.

Nursing homes that do participate in the Medicare program are often referred to as Skilled Nursing Facilities (SNF). They have a strong financial base for providing rehabilitation services to qualified patients since they pass the cost of those rehabilitation services to Medicare. The nursing home administrator needs to understand this financial benefit and clearly appreciate his options before deciding not to participate in the Medicare program.

QUALITY SERVICES

Once the elderly individual has entered a Skilled Nursing Facility, there are no assurances that he or she will receive quality rehabilitation. There are many example of why. Many SNFs provide only a fragment of the total services required (the Medicare laws do not require that all rehabilitation services be provided). Often only nursing or only nursing and physical therapy is provided to an individual who may also need speech and occupational therapy. Also, some therapists consult with as many as 12 or 15 nursing homes. They are spread so thin that as a practical matter the patient will receive less therapy than the therapists themselves would agree is needed. Finally, there are circumstances in which team members do not effectively communicate. An example of this can be seen in the documentation of services when one team member documents independence in an activity such as dressing and another team member documents a need for cueing and minimal assist in dressing for the same patient. This can result in a denial of payment for those services.

Create a Rehabilitation Team

The consumer has the right to expect all necessary therapies in a coordinated fashion and at a frequency and duration that will produce the rehabilitation effect. To maximize the chance of providing coordinated, quality rehabilitation, therapists need to work as a team (Maguire, 1985). Each discipline has a unique and invaluable contribution to make in the rehabilitation process. Nursing or occupational therapy alone, however, will not be able to succeed in most cases. Furthermore, the team needs a "coach," someone who is able to see the broad picture and to help the team appropriately allocate its resources. If an effective team leader exists in your building, support that person. When one does not exist, provide that coordination yourself. If this is not possible because of your schedule or other reasons, seek out another member of the team, express your interest in him or her being a team leader and offer your genuine support.

Educate

One of your most potent team building strategies is education. Take every opportunity to teach administrators, directors of nursing and other staff the importance and effectiveness of working as a team. Invite the administrator and director of nursing to attend your inservices. Cite positive examples of how the nursing staff, in cooperation with other rehabilitation services, was instrumental in sending a patient home fully independent in dressing, for example.

Set the Example

Whenever you have the opportunity, set an example. When in the staff break room or at the nurse's station, speak positively about team members. When there are schedule conflicts with nursing or other rehabilitation providers, help to problem solve so that all parties are winners. Win-win solutions to problems help create and nurture the team approach to patient care. Generally, it is best to praise in public and criticize in private. When an aide or other team member performs well, praise her or him in front of peers. Be balanced in that approach and find something good to praise in all the team members. Collaborate with members of the team to provide solutions to problems such as patient management. Help team members remember that the patient is the focus and reason for the team's existence.

Establish Lines of Communications

In settings where there are none, initiate weekly rehabilitation meetings to discuss the patients' progress toward their rehabilitation goals. To overcome the initial resistance to such a meeting, find an ally to help lobby for the meeting. Establish simple ground rules that will prevent the waste of precious time. For example, spend no more than 10 minutes on each patient. The meeting should last only 30 minutes if you are discussing three patients. Meet at the same time and place each week to maximize attendance. Finally, the nursing aides should be active participants in these meetings. They have an important perspective of the patient to share.

Once a weekly rehabilitation meeting is established and has proven its value, suggest to the administrator that potential patients be briefly discussed at this meeting. This is especially useful when there are limited rehabilitation beds in your facility and there is a waiting list of potential patients. This approach minimizes the chances of either overlooking or overestimating the patients' rehabilitation potential.

CONCLUSION

The population growth of those 65 years and older will have far reaching consequences on our health care system and, of special concern to therapists, on rehabilitation of the aged. Our challenge as rehabilitation specialists is to broaden our role to become rehabilitation advocates. As rehabilitation advocates we must be leaders in improving access to rehabilitation services, in informing other health care providers of the value of rehabilitation and in assuring that these rehabilitation services are of the highest quality.

REFERENCES

Johnson, B. Jr.: Marketing Rehabilitation Services: Buying and Selling Effectively. *Topics in Geriatric Rehabilitation*, 1987, 2(2),37-45.
Levenson, S.A.: Innovations in Nursing Home Care. *Generations,* 1987, 12(1), 74-79.

Maguire, G.H.: The team approach in action. In Maguire, G.H. (Ed.): *Care of the Elderly: A Health Team Approach*. Boston. Little, Brown & Company, 1985.

National Center for Health Statistics, P. M. Golden: *Charting the Nation's Health: Trends Since 1960*. DHHS Pub. No. (PHS) 85-1251. Public Health Service, Washington, DC. U.S. Government Printing Office, August, 1985.

President's Commission for the Study of Ethical Problems in Medicine and Biomedical and Behavioral Research: *Securing Access to Health Care: The Ethical Implications of the Differences in the Availability of Health Services*, Volume 1. Washington DC. U.S. Government Printing Office, March, 1983.

Riche, M. F.: The Nursing Home Dilemma. *American Demographics*, October, 1985, 35-39.

Schick, F. L. (Ed.): *Statistical Handbook on Aging Americans*. Phoenix, Arizona. The Onyx Press, 1986.

Technological Applications
to Promote Independent Living
in the Elderly

Jeanne Ryan, MA, OTR
Anne Marie Werner, MA, OTR
Judith Wasserman Lipton, MA, OTR

Current estimates are that 10,000 Spinal Cord injuries occur annually (King & Dudas, 1986). For every million persons in the country there are 35 injuries with a total of 200,000 persons in the United States with a spinal cord injury at this time (Young, 1976). The National Spinal Cord Registry reported that 40% of Spinal Cord injuries are caused by vehicular accidents, 20% are caused by falls and 40% are caused by gunshot wounds, sporting accidents, industrial accidents and agricultural accidents in order of decreasing importance (Bennethum, 1981). Approximately 85% of Spinal Cord injuries are sustained by males during the peak age range of 18-28 years (Hardy & Elson, 1976). Rehabilitation of the Spinal Cord injured patient is lengthy, requiring 100-160 days for a paraplegic and 180-300 days for a quadriplegic (Panchal, 1978).

Although the individuals most at risk for incurring a spinal cord injury are teenaged and young adult males, the improved life expectancy of the elderly has resulted in an increasing number of middle-aged and elderly spinal cord injured persons. This article is chiefly concerned with the latter population.

As our society ages, the number of older persons is expected to double by the year 2030. In 1980, people over 65 represented 11.3%

Jeanne Ryan, Senior Occupational Therapist, Anne Marie Werner, Staff Occupational Therapist, and Judith Wasserman Lipton, Chief Occupational Therapist, Goldwater Memorial Hospital, Roosevelt Island, New York, NY 10044.

of the total U.S. population, or every ninth person. Between 1970 and 1980 this older population grew by 28%. Every day about 5,200 Americans celebrate their sixty-fifth birthday, and approximately 3,600 persons over age 65 die, for a net increase of 1,600 older Americans daily. Nearly 75% of those who reach 65 years of age will live past 75 (U.S. Special Subcommittee on Aging, 1984).

Although a review of the literature did not reveal a reliable breakdown of geriatric spinal cord injured persons, it is becoming increasingly clear that the institutionalization of older adults is often the result of a spinal injury. For example, of the 24 spinal cord injured persons admitted to Goldwater Memorial Hospital's Respiratory unit, 14 were over 55 years of age.

Goldwater Memorial Hospital is a 912 bed facility with Rehabilitation, Medicine and Skilled Nursing Units. A long-term care facility for the severely disabled, Goldwater houses the Howard A. Rusk Respiratory Center. Although the spinal injuries were from different causes (motor vehicle accident, polio) all presented with the same diagnosis: quadriplegia. These numbers include only patients admitted to one rehabilitation unit and do not reflect the large number of admissions to our Skilled Nursing facility.

ROLE OF THE OCCUPATIONAL THERAPIST

Although specific treatment varies depending upon the level of injury, occupational therapy intervention usually includes range of motion, strengthening and endurance exercises, progressive wheelchair sitting, functional activities and vocational assessment. Rehabilitation of the geriatric spinal cord injured person requires many specialized services to optimize function. The following case study illustrates the special considerations in rehabilitation of this population.

Background Information

L.M. was a self sufficient woman living on her own, who fell during the night while getting up to eat. At 72 she was working as a housekeeper, which she had done since coming to New York in 1946. At the time of her admission to Goldwater Memorial Hospital she presented with C5-C6 quadriplegia, was dependent in all self care, severely limited in range of motion of both upper extremities and was unable to sit unsupported. A treatment plan was formulated which included wheelchair positioning, active range of motion activities, muscle strengthening exercises and ADL independence including power wheelchair mobility, feeding, grooming and leisure interests.

And So It Begins

When L.M. entered Goldwater Memorial Hospital she came from an acute care hospital where she had been in bed for a month. The first and most important goal was to get her properly positioned in a wheelchair. Once this was accomplished she could progress to power wheelchair training and self care skills. Assessment and provision of specialized equipment proved to be lengthy series of trial and error. She came to the Occupational Therapy clinic on a stretcher but transferred to a wheelchair during her treatment to try different approaches to her seating problems. Many different combinations of equipment were tried. A solid seat, an angled seat, a lapboard, but she never looked right. Every day she went back to the unit on the stretcher. Her therapist felt a sense of failure, promising to find the solution tomorrow. L.M. always ended those treatment sessions saying she was in no hurry, that we were doing our best.

As therapist and patient struggled to find the solution to her seating problem she told me that she had left her family in South Carolina to come to New York. She was the second eldest of nine children and wanted to make enough money to help her brothers and sisters through school (an opportunity she herself had passed up). While on the stretcher she would practice her active range of motion with the assistance of the deltoid aid. Often while swinging her arms into horizontal abduction she would describe the farm where she grew up. She was a very physical woman, she had been all her life. When asked about now being paralyzed she said she had had a good life, only now she would be in a chair. There was a peaceful acceptance to L.M. which was not always understandable, but greatly appreciated as this allowed us to work at our own pace, trying new things and learning what would and wouldn't work. With the help of the more experienced therapists, we were able to find the right equipment.

Because she lacked sufficient trunk balance and hip flexion to sit independently in a wheelchair, L.M. required extensive positioning equipment to maintain an upright position. She was provided with an angled seat which afforded her 90° of hip flexion (Figure 1). Additionally, a solid back with lateral trunk supports prevented her from falling to one side (Figure 2). Hip guides were provided to maintain her hips in a neutral position (Figure 3). She had bilateral foot drop which necessitated a specially designed footboard to maintain her feet in a neutral position (Figure 4). Lastly, L.M. was provided with a lapboard to improve upper extremity symmetry and

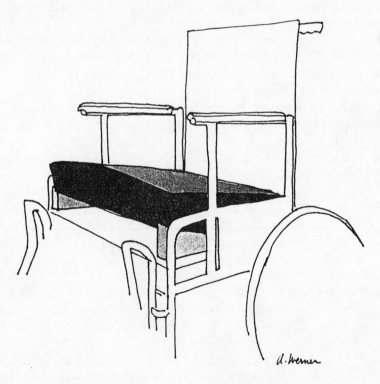

Figure 1

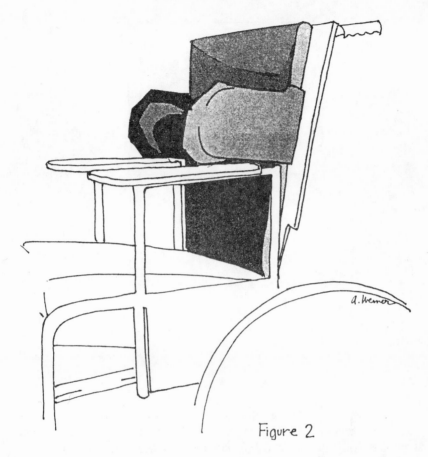

Figure 2

provide her with a surface for eating (Figure 5). Bilateral resting splints allowed her to maintain her hands in a functional position as she had no active wrist movement and very little finger movement.

The Next Step

A power wheelchair was ordered with a chin control set-up. Due to her upper extremity limitations, this seemed to be the only appropriate method of power mobility. When the wheelchair arrived in the clinic, L.M. was very upset at the prospect of having a large box in front of her face. How could she talk to her friends and the staff?

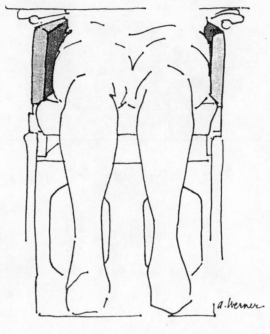

Figure 3

How could she show off her hairstyles (courtesy of the nursing staff)? No one would be able to see her face. Although her concerns were understandable, a quick solution to our problems was not forthcoming. As a therapist with all of six months experience there appeared to be no other way for her to drive her chair. L.M. insisted she could drive the chair with her hand.

With some skepticism on the part of the therapist, we agreed to give it a try. Initially, the joystick was mounted to the lapboard and an overhead sling was attached to her chair to allow her to drive with her right hand. Since she had no wrist or hand movements, she would be driving with her shoulder and elbow musculature. L.M. wore an ADL cuff to stabilize her wrist and forearm. She tried to hook the joystick with the ADL cuff and drive with the assistance of the overhead sling. At the end of two weeks she suggested that we get rid of the overhead sling since this gave her too much mobility

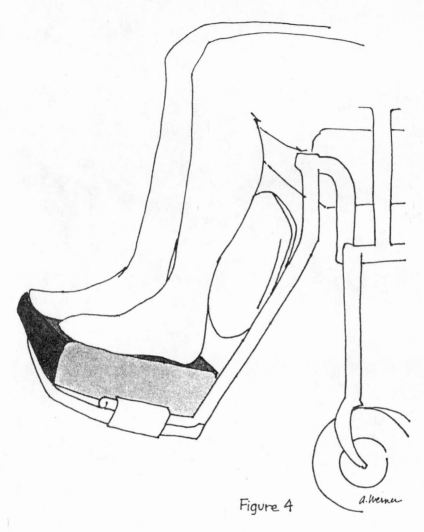

Figure 4

and not enough control. Without the sling she could drive the chair forward using shoulder protraction/flexion and elbow extension and backwards using shoulder retraction/extension and elbow flexion. With this small amount of success we were both convinced that we could find a way. During that week we tried many different types of joysticks without success. What was needed was a way to use

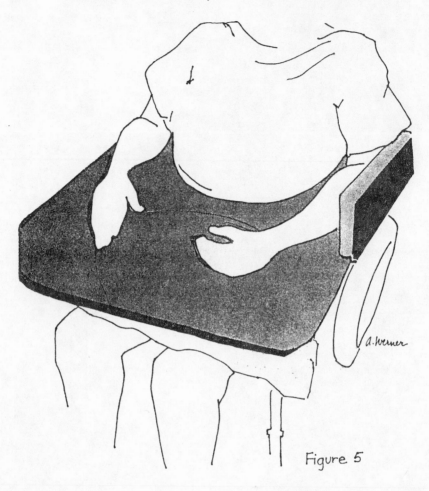

Figure 5

shoulder internal rotation to turn left and external rotation to turn right. With the active involvement of L.M. we found a way to fasten her hand to the joystick and fabricated her present method control.

A Method to Our Madness

Using aquaplast, a U-Bar the length of her hand was screwed into the top of a very small joystick (Figure 6). It fit snugly enough to stabilize her hand and at the same time allowed the movements at

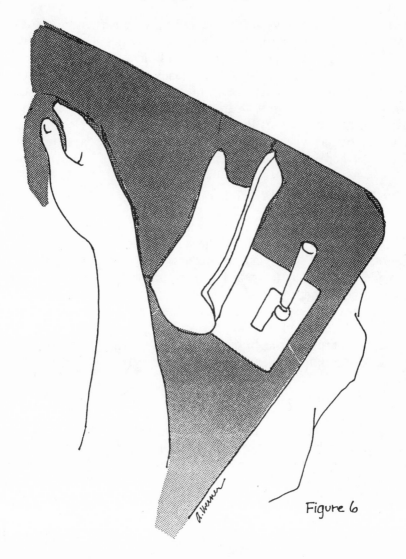

Figure 6

her shoulder to do the driving. During the next month she practiced driving straight, making right and left turns, negotiating doorways and small spaces and entering and exiting the elevator. A cylindrical tube was placed on top of the on/off switch and by hooking her ADL cuff on this she was able to independently turn the chair on and off. Once L.M. was independently driving her wheelchair she was able to participate in many hospital activities. Goldwater is a very large hospital, much larger in length than height. An average worker or ambulatory patient could easily walk a mile in one day just getting from place to place. L.M. was now able to attend chapel when she wished, visit with friends and participate in the maintenance of her wheelchair. Patients are able to drive to Occupational Therapy or the wheelchair repair shop when there is a problem. This gave her some control over her life.

Moving on from There

From this point L.M. easily learned to feed herself using a fork positioned in her ADL cuff and the same motions she used to drive the wheelchair. With a plate stabilized to her lapboard, she used her shoulder movements to spear her food, and her biceps and triceps enabled her to get the food from her plate to her mouth. With the help of her ADL splints, she was able to use an evenflo cup for drinking. With an adapted toothbrush also placed in her splint she was able to brush her teeth, using head movement to substitute for her lack of arm movement.

Seeing It Through Together

Throughout her eight months of treatment L.M. was an active participant in her therapy. I learned to listen to her, trusting she knew her body. As an older individual she came to rehab with the patience for change that her younger therapist lacked. She brought vitality to our department and taught me the value of persevering.

REFERENCES

Bennethum, S.E. Spinal Cord Injury. In B. Abreu (Ed.), Physical Disabilities Manual. New York: Raven, 1981.

Hardy, A., and Elson, R. Practical Management of Spinal Cord Injuries. New York: Churchill Livingstone, 1976.

King, R.B. and Dudas, S. Rehabilitation of the patient with a spinal injury. *Nursing Clin. North America*, 1986, 15, 225-243.

McKenzie, M.W. and Buck, G. L. Combined motor and peripheral insufficiency: Management of spinal cord injury. *Phys. Ther.*, 1978, 58, 294-303.

Panchal, P.D., Rehabilitation of the patient with a spinal cord injury. *Prog. Surg.*, 1978, 16, 207-220.

U.S. Senate, Special Committee on Aging and Am. Assoc. of Retired Persons, "Aging America: Trends and Projections" Washington DC: U.S. Govt Printing Office, 1984.

The Wheelchair:
An Adult Scooter Board

Estelle B. Breines, PhD, OTR, FAOTA

SUMMARY. Although the treatment concept of sensory integration was developed to serve the needs of learning disabled children, its principles were adapted to meet the needs of adults. However, therapeutic tools used with children can be unsatisfactory when used with adults, particularly the elderly, because they are apt to be characterized as toys. This paper analyzes the effects of propulsive linear mobility on neural, perceptual and functional performance and proposes that the wheelchair provides similar therapeutic functions for adults as does the scooter board for children.

INTRODUCTION

Sensory integration (SI) treatment is based in part on the premise that vestibular stimulation effects integration of the sensory systems (Ayres, 1972a). The assumption that movement through space can be therapeutic serves as a foundation for treatment, and is the basis for many of the tools and activities designed to generate this integration.

SI principles and practices originally were developed to aid in the resolution of children's learning disorders. Learning disorders were viewed to be neural in origin, stemming from disorders in the maturation of the nervous system. As these principles, and the treatment techniques that were developed from these principles, were observed to be effective in resolving children's learning disorders,

Estelle B. Breines is President, Geri-Rehab, Inc., Executive Director, Developmental Re/habilitation Services, 170 Hibbler Road, Lebanon, NJ 08833, and Clinical Assistant Professor, Department of Occupational Therapy, New York University.

25

therapists began to use similar techniques with other populations. Thus, SI concepts were expanded to include adult populations with mental and physical disorders.

This translation of a treatment modality from one realm of practice to another created some problems. One problem is that the SI evaluation techniques, albeit subject to some criticism (Yerxa, 1982), are standardized on a youthful population. Despite Petersen, Goar and Van Deusen's (1985) attempt to rectify this short fall by acquiring some baseline data on adults, comprehensive norms have not been established for adult populations. Therefore, treatment offered to adults is not founded on scientific demonstration of need according to the same parameters as the population upon which the *Southern California Sensory Integration Tests* (Ayres, 1972b) were developed. Secondly, some practitioners use the term sensory integration when referring to sensory stimulation that is not necessarily provided by movement. Since certification in SI is granted to those demonstrating competency with children, these therapists tend to be more accurate in using SI terminology than therapists who treat adults exclusively. These considerations probably contribute to the fact that SI treatment of the adult has not been fully analyzed or justified. Despite these considerations, occupational therapists state they use SI treatments with adults with varying diagnoses (King, 1974; Ross and Burdyck, 1981).

To contribute to the body of knowledge regarding the use of SI treatment techniques with adults, this paper attempts to demonstrate that similar concepts are valid for children and adults, that self-induced linear or propulsive movement enables the integration of sensory stimuli, and that the wheelchair and the scooter board are similar in providing that stimulation.

SENSORY INTEGRATION WITH ADULTS

SI treatment for adults has been discussed by two primary sources. King (1974), first to discuss the role of sensory integration in the treatment of adults, proposed its use with chronic schizophrenic patients. Generalized movement was recommended to enhance sensory stimulation, and a variety of activities were designed to incorporate movement into the treatment regimen. Ross and Burdyck (1981), describing SI treatment of confused elderly patients, advocated the use of vestibular stimulation techniques (p. 4). In addition to describing activities which require generalized movement, they suggested the use of the scooter board for treatment (p. 20), and adapted techniques initially used with children for use with adults. However, the movement techniques described are primarily rotary in character. While propulsive scooter board activities are customarily used as treatment for children to enhance the integration of vestibular, tactual, visual and other neural stimulation, the use of propulsive movement techniques for adults is not discussed. Analysis of the movement aspects of SI treatment of adults appears to have been restricted to the discussion of generalized movement and passive and active rotary techniques, whereas treatment of children has been discussed by Ayres both in terms of rotary and linear movement stimulation.

CONSIDERATIONS OF AGING

The integration of sensory stimuli from a variety of sensors is requisite to performance and to orientation. Such orientation is developed as a course of normal development. Yet, the sensory systems of the elderly are subject to decline (Corso, 1971; Breines, 1980), often making previously developed skills nonfunctional. Since the elderly are subject to visual and auditory deficits and losses in tactile function and proprioception, patients with such deficits are sometimes disoriented. This phenomenon is described in terms of many diagnoses and is attributed to different sources, but may be described universally as sensory disintegration. Therefore, despite diagnosis, SI is relevant treatment for patients with perceptual disorders manifested as disorientation, confusion, dyspraxia, and memory disorders.

One reason for the dearth of propulsive mobility activities designed for adults may be that toys and games designed for use with children are not ordinarily successful tools for adults. Although clinicians may be using elongated scooter boards such as Ross and Burdyck describe, these activities are not customarily adult activities particularly for the aged who compose a considerable segment of the adult disabled population. Aside from the potential hazard of such activity, adults, young and old, able and disabled, are often unwilling to engage in childish activities. In addition, the physical weight of disabled adults needs to be considered. The need to transfer patients to and from the floor for scooter board activities tends to limit their practicality for adults, particularly those who are multiply handicapped. This limitation is especially noted in facilities which do not have appropriate space, equipment, or personnel, or view these types of mobility activities as inappropriate for adults. However, such restrictions do not necessarily limit opportunities for propulsive mobility. Propulsion can easily be effected by use of the wheelchair.

WHEELCHAIR TRAINING AS A THERAPEUTIC TOOL

Extensive clinical experience with disabled elderly patients reveals that wheelchair training has often been instrumental in restoring orientation in elderly patients with a variety of diagnoses commonly associated with aging (Breines, 1981). Such results led the author to recognize similarities between the wheelchair and the scooter board commonly used in SI practice. Their similarity in linear mobility has been analyzed, and it is suggested that the theories which substantiate SI practice may hold true for the treatment of adults as well.

Occupational therapy treatment often includes practical training of patients in life skills along with neural stimulation techniques. Instructing patients in the use of the wheelchair can serve a number of purposes. Wheelchair mobility is generally acknowledged to be a functional skill. This paper presents the wheelchair as a tool that offers neural stimulation and perceptual reorganization along with functional mobility.

Wheelchairs should be individually fitted, adapted and retained by the patient for whom the chair is intended. Patients should be instructed in wheelchair use in the broadest perspective of propulsion and way-finding in order to provide therapy in several realms simultaneously. Although I have occasionally put ambulatory patients into wheelchairs to effect the changes suggested in this paper, for the most part, the use of the wheelchair as a therapeutic tool is recommended for the patient for whom the wheelchair is a necessary tool for transit.

LINEAR MOBILITY AS THERAPY

The wheelchair is not ordinarily thought of as an SI tool. Rather, it is generally considered a transport tool. Yet, these are not dissimilar concepts. Transportation provides vestibular stimulation as well as stimulation to other sensors. If movement is self-induced and meets the goals or needs of the patient, one can conclude, as has Trombly (1982), its effectiveness in sensory-motoric therapy. Since both scooter boards and wheelchairs offer stimulation and orientation effects from the linear or propulsive movement they provide and the success experience they enable, they can be understood to be similar in purpose.

Wheelchairs and scooter boards are tools that enable and reinforce self-induced forward propulsion. During propulsion, multiple sensory systems receive simultaneous stimulation. Yet, simultaneous stimulation does not assure that individuals perceive their environment accurately, nor that function is enabled. Rather, it is the integration of the perception of time and space that enables function. (Breines, 1981, 1986a, 1986b). Such integration requires repeated experience in meaningful situations. Performance requires the accurate synthesis or integration of senses that monitor mobility through time and space in order for functional experience to be perceived.

In describing SI theory, Cool (1987) emphasizes the role of the motor systems in integrating the sensory systems, leading us to understand that between and within each sensory system, sensorimotor components must function in an integrated manner for the unified perception of action in time and space to result. Therefore, the integration of sensation and the integration of the perception of time and space can be viewed as two sides of the same coin. SI can be understood to be both a neurological and a perceptual phenomenon. Actually, there is no empirical evidence for the integration of sensation as a neural phenomenon. Rather, integration is assumed, based on the observation of performance and interpretations of perception. While integration is discussed in terms of neural function, the assumption underlying the use of the scooter board is that, over time, the sensory and motor stimulation afforded by linear propulsion, along with other treatments, enables sensory data to be perceived in an integrated fashion.

Function requires both neural and perceptual integration. Integration is the resolution of temporal/spatial discrepancies (Breines, 1981, 1986a, 1986b). This potential for discrepancy can be understood, for example, in terms of the visual system. In linear movement, the peripheral field is afforded a more rapidly changing display than the frontal field. As one propels through the environment, one is stimulated by a multiplicity of laterally located objects and spaces, whereas frontal vision remains focused on the center of the field. The only marked change in the frontal field is the increased dimension of the goal object as the individual nears it. This change pales by comparison with the variety of rapidly changing stimuli assaulting the peripheral fields. Peripheral field inputs serve to orient frontal data (Rock, 1975). The disparity between frontal and peripheral visual stimuli is synthesized or integrated, resolving the differential between front and side dimensions, providing a mechanism for orientation, and subserving function (Breines, 1981).

Gibson (1970) informs us that frontal and peripheral vision circuits to different brain centers along different neural tracts. Ambient or peripheral vision circuits to the superior colliculus; foveal or central vision circuits to the cortex. Because these loci differ, there is a potential differential in speed of processing and level of neural function. Therefore, peripheral and foveal interpretations of space may differ, or be unreliable, contributing to confusion and disorientation. A resolution of this differential is required for performance to be reliable. In normal development this resolution takes place in infancy. Such resolution remains functional throughout life unless acquired disability results and immobilization occurs, as is frequently demonstrated by the institutionalized elderly. One must recall that visual deficits of the elderly may be peripheral or foveal in nature, and along with immobilization can interfere with perception and orientation.

Propulsive mobility provides other stimulation and experience as well. Using wheelchairs and scooter boards requires upper extremity motoric patterns in which the proprioceptors in the joints and muscles of the arms, shoulders, and trunk are stimulated. While use of the scooter board stimulates the hands by contact with the ground, the hands also receive stimulation from wheelchair rims. But in either case, it is the resisted movement of the arms through space that allows the mover to perceive distance. Whether the hands directly touch the ground, or indirectly relate to the ground through the wheel, they are oriented to spatial change through the proprioceptive system in conjunction with the visual and vestibular systems.

Just as early development establishes orientation by propulsion through space, reorientation has these same requirements. It may be that earliest orientation develops through the mobility of the upper extremities, which precedes that of the lowers. If so, this might explain why wheelchair training is orienting and ambulation appears to be less so. The integrated use of upper extremities, vision, hearing, and vestibular function may be the foundational mechanism for spatial organization and thus, orientation. According to Cool (1987), the vestibular system is the neural system that organizes other sensory systems, but it may be upper extremity proprioceptors that ground the vestibular system in space, and the visual system that confirms it through feedback. However, the issue of upper or lower extremities may be moot. The use of the wheelchair as an orienting tool may be mandatory, for many patients are limited in independent ambulation, and the wheelchair provides them opportunities otherwise unavailable.

Integration of sensory-motoric elements in purposeful mobility contributes to the stability and orientation necessary for function, and provides a mechanism for spatial orientation. Directionality and distance, the aspects by which space is known, are reinforced by the purposeful use of mobility tools. This phenomenon is in constant operation throughout life in new situations and is a feature of human adaptation. It would appear that since spatial orientation and sensory integration can be developed in later years, this developmental phenomenon could be instrumental in reorienting disabled adults.

Just as children experience success in scooter board activities and are gratified by their play, the wheelchair is a functional and reinforcing tool for adults. Both tools reinforce the perception of space through opportunities for success experience. Forward propulsion and accurate turns to right and left lead to success in achieving meaningful goals. In addition to the below conscious or "sub-cortical" integration of neural inputs that is presumed to occur with movement, deliberate sighting of locations and using those locations as goal objects enable patients to orient to their surround, and to participate in meaningful activities. Careful grading of controlled distances, locations, and objectives, from the familiar to the unfamiliar, from small increments to large, leads to increased orientation and independence in mobility. This in turn leads to increased self-confidence, and risk-taking in further exploration.

The use of meaningful tools in the performance of life's tasks is acknowledged to enhance function. It should not be surprising that meaningful tools can differ for adults and children, while providing similar stimulation and integration, and meeting similar needs. Therefore, although the motoric requirements of wheelchairs and scooter boards are not identical, they are sufficiently similar to be used in similar ways, while meeting the socially appropriate needs and goals of age specific populations.

CONCLUSION

This paper has presented the view that SI principles of value to the child can also be of value to the adult; however, the tools of childhood are not the tools of the adult. Adults and children find meaning in different activities; therefore, their tools differ. The wheelchair and the scooter board are both tools which permit self-initiated propulsive mobility, but meet different goal needs of adults and children.

The use of these tools has been analyzed from the perspective that linear or propulsive mobility provides the neural *and* perceptual systems with the opportunity to resolve temporal/spatial discrepancies, a concept compatible with that of SI. It has been suggested that this resolution or integration underlies orientation and thus function. Therefore, tools that enable function differ according to patients' preferences, because patients' needs are more likely to be met when treatment is structured by self-initiated goals to move. Tools that provide mobility in ways that meet the differing styles of children and adults enable them to meet their own goals.

Occupational therapists commonly analyze principles and tools found valuable in one area of practice, and translate and adapt these for use with other populations. This is one more instance in which concepts developed for and successful in one area of practice have been adapted and analyzed in such a way as to address the needs of another population.

REFERENCES

Ayres, AJ. *Sensory Integration and Learning Disorders*. Los Angeles, Western Psychological: 1972a.

Ayres, AJ. *Southern California Sensory Integration Tests*. Los Angeles, Western Psychological: 1972b.

Breines, E. *Perceptual Changes in Aging*. Lebanon, NJ, Geri-Rehab: 1980.

Breines, E. *Perception: Its Development and Recapitulation*. Lebanon, NJ, Geri-Rehab: 1981.

Breines, E. *Origins and Adaptations: A Philosophy of Practice*. Lebanon, NJ, Geri-Rehab: 1986a; Pragmatism, A Philosophical Foundation of Occupational Therapy, 1900-1922 and 1968-1985; Implications for Specialization and Education. PhD dissertation, New York University, 1986b.

Cool, SJ. A View from the "Outside": Sensory Integration and Developmental Neurobiology. *Sensory Integration Special Interest Section Newsletter* 10, 2: 2,3, 1987.

Corso, J. Sensory Processes and Age Effects in Normal Adults. *Journal of Gerontology* 26: 9-105, 1971.

Gibson, E. The development of perception as an adaptive process. *American Scientist* 58, 1970: 98-107.

King, LJ. A sensory integrative approach to schizophrenia. *American Journal of Occupational Therapy* 28 (October 1974): 529-536.

Petersen, P Goar, D & Van Deusen, J. Performance of female adults on the Southern California Visual Figure Ground Perception Test. *American Journal of Occupational Therapy* 39 (August 1985): 525-530.

Rock, I. *An Introduction to Perception*. New York: Macmillan: 1975.

Ross, M & Burdyck, D. *Sensory Integration: A Training Manual for Therapists and Teachers for Regressed Psychiatric and Geriatric Patient Groups*. Thorofare, NJ, Charles B. Slack: 1981

Trombly, CA. Include exercise in "purposeful activity." *American Journal of Occupational Therapy*, 36 (July 1982): 467-468.

Yerxa, E. The Issue: A response to testing and measurement in occupational therapy: A review of current practice with special emphasis on the Southern California Sensory Integration Tests. *American Journal of Occupational Therapy* 36 (June 1982): 399-404.

The Effects of Touch in the Geriatric Population

Deborah M. Howard

SUMMARY. The current study investigated the effects of touch in a population of nursing home residents. Thirty individuals were randomly chosen to participate in a craft session. Sixteen participants were touched while fourteen were not touched. Participants completed a questionnaire immediately after the craft session. Responses to the questionnaire were statistically analyzed by means of chi square. Results found that tactile stimulation positively impacts attitude and motivation in the elderly. The touch group participants indicated strong, positive responses regarding attitude toward the task and the instructor. The touch group showed greater willingness to work for the instructor and complete a task. Touching is a positive influence on the geriatric person's attitudes and behaviors toward both a task and therapist. More sensitive instruments are needed to determine the relationship between touch and mood since it was not significant in this study.

INTRODUCTION

The effects of a simple touch are considered vital to human function. Yet, little empirical exploration has been conducted in the area of occupational therapy with respect to touch. The current study was designed to examine, in the aged population, the effect of touch

Research submitted by Deborah M. Howard has been approved and accepted in partial fulfillment of the requirements for the degree of Master of Occupational Therapy from the University of Puget Sound.

The author would like to thank the following people for their individual contributions toward making this paper a reality: Juli Evans, MS, OTR/L, Steven Morelan, PhD, OTR/L, Ron Stone, MS, OTR/L, and Thomas Sharon, Administrator, Sharon Guest Home.

35

on patients' behaviors and attitudes regarding both a task and the treating therapist.

The issue of touch has been controversial in the therapeutic setting. Twenty-five years ago, it was considered taboo for a therapist to touch a client, while today a casual touch is considered appropriate and helpful (Cohen, Lotyczewski, & Weissberg, 1982). "Clinical literature points to therapeutic potential of touch in nearly every branch of medicine from psychiatry to gerontology" (Older, 1984, p. 931). Modern day health professionals may choose to use touch as a powerful tool for communicating their caring (Pertillo, 1978) as touch can affect an individual's behavior and affective state.

Touch is the giving and receiving of tactile stimulation. A touch on the shoulder or hand is universal, common, and non-sexual in connotation (Anderton & Heckel, 1985; Fisher & Whitcher, 1979; Rosenfield & Sussman, 1978). Three conditions can make a touch positive: (a) appropriateness to the situation, (b) appropriate degree of intimacy as perceived by the recipient, and (c) lack of a negative or condescending message (Fisher & Whitcher, 1979). As stated by Heslin and Patterson (1982), ". . . a casual touch by a stranger can be more positive than negative, and it has the power to influence a person's general sense of well-being" (p. 36). An appropriate touch can convey a positive message to the recipient.

Patients are often more aware of a health professional's concern, caring, and confidence than the touch itself (Farber, 1982; Huss, 1977; & Montagu, 1978). "The fact we are not aware of most tactile input does not mean that is not important. . . . If the brain is deprived of touch stimulation, it very quickly becomes disorganized" (Ayres, 1979, p. 96). Increased awareness of touch by the occupational therapist can help decrease the psychological barriers between the patient and therapist and improve therapist-client relationships in general.

Traditionally, touch has been acknowledged as a tool to enhance communication (Frith & Lindsey, 1983). Communication through touch has increased compliance levels of petition signing, retrieving dropped pamphlets, returning dimes left in telephone booths, and even eating free grocery store food (Fordyce & Goldman, 1983 & Kleinke, 1977). Fordyce and Goldman (1983) justified the compliance phenomenon by saying,

> Having eye contact from or being touched by a requester may lead to more compliance because the requester is viewed as psychologically closer to the target person, or is more individualized, or because the target person is more aware of the requester's needs. (p. 126)

Communication is an essential component of occupational therapy. Verbal, visual, and tactile communication increase the potential for patient response and compliance. A casual touch may increase compliance levels in patients who are unmotivated by or uninterested in projects presented to them.

Tactile stimulation increases compliance as well as other positive behaviors and attitudes during therapy. Individuals touched during counseling sessions readily talked about themselves and evaluated the interview and the interviewer as being more positive (Alagna, Fisher, Whitcher, & Wicas, 1979 & Pattison, 1973). Using touch as the basic technique in treating geriatric patients with chronic brain syndrome, Burnside (1973) found the group behaved more amiably and reached out to touch one another more frequently. Within the realm of occupational therapy, Eyler (1983), found touch had a positive effect on participant attitudes toward individual performance, the activity, and the instructor.

The elderly are often deprived of human contact. Pertillo (1978) offers two explanations for this phenomenon. First, many people refrain from touching older individuals because they may possess unpleasant physical characteristics (Pertillo, 1978). Second, the elderly population displays more inhibitions about touching due to limitations dictated to them by society (Pertillo, 1978).

Personal space, body language, and dialogue are clues contributing to the therapist's perceptual awareness of each gerontic client's need for tactile stimulation. Some clues are louder than others.

> As I held her hand with its tissue paper skin, she pulled my head down to her and kissed me tenderly on the cheek. . . . This was the best example of "touch hunger" I had seen in a long while. (Burnside, 1973 p. 2060)

Often, as individuals reach "old age," they begin to rely on the non-verbal behaviors they learned during younger years (Huss,

1977 & Preston, 1973). Huss (1977) found many elderly persons handle sentimental material objects, such as a wedding ring or picture of a deceased spouse. Although little research has been done in the gerontic setting, touch could be an important tool in therapeutically maintaining the health of the aged.

Fisher and Whitcher (1979) implied that touch may have consequences for behavior and affective state. Behaviorally, touch seems to facilitate compliance. Compliance is needed for adequate client response and, possibly, motivation. Affective response has been found to be positive if a touch is considered appropriate by the recipient. Touch in the gerontic setting has not been investigated. Presumably, both behavior and affective states would be altered as with other populations studied.

Awareness of the implications and advantages of touch used in the gerontic setting may be helpful to all allied health professionals. Specific awareness of touch and its effects on the elderly individual may be crucial to occupational therapy treatment. This study examined the effect of touch on the elderly person's attitude and the resultant motivation toward an activity and the therapist. Finally, the effect of touch on mood state was examined.

METHOD

Subjects

Thirty females age 65 and over were selected using the following specific criteria: the capacity to follow written or verbal instructions and to attend to the task, and the absence of any upper extremity deficit which would interfere with completion of the task. The subjects were randomly selected from an all female nursing home population, then randomly divided into six groups. Members of three groups received tactile stimulation while those of the other three groups did not.

Materials and Tests

A large room which accommodated ten or more people, wheelchairs, and a large table, and which provided plenty of natural light was used. During the first part of the session, verbal instructions were given to construct a bookmark using felt, glue, and scissors. A questionnaire was administered during the second part of the session. Five response areas were identified by the author as potentially affected by touch after three pilot studies. The response categories were (a) attitude toward the instructor, (b) mood before, during, and after the craft session, (c) attitude toward the task itself (d) motivation to work on the project, and (e) motivation to work for the instructor. Items made strong statements and were written in the first person. Subjects were asked to circle the response they judged most appropriate. The response choices were the same throughout the questionnaire: strongly agree, agree, disagree, and strongly disagree (see Appendix A).

Procedures

Each group met with the same instructor who gave verbal instructions for performing the activity (see Appendix B). After the directions were given, the instructor offered advice and encouragement regarding the assembly of the bookmark. "Can I help you?", "Good job!", and "How are you doing?" were acceptable comments. Subjects were not encouraged to make another bookmark or leave the room. In the no-touch groups, the instructor spoke but did not touch the subjects. In the touch groups, the instructor spoke and lightly touched each subject on the shoulder. Each touch lasted approximately four seconds, and individuals were touched between four and eight times during the activity. The length and amount of contact were determined as a result of three pilot studies. The specific form of contact used in this study was chosen because it was deemed to be non-threatening to the participants. Depending on the fine motor dexterity of the participants the entire craft project took between 20 and 40 minutes to complete. Upon finishing the project, each individual completed the questionnaire. If a participant was unable to read or write, the questionnaire was administered verbally and the responses recorded. Nine participants, five from the touch group and four from the no-touch group, were unable to read or write.

RESULTS

Subjects in the touch group reported stronger and more positive judgements in response to all questionnaire statements than did the no-touch group subjects. This difference was found to be statistically significant using a Chi Square (χ^2 (1, N = 89) = 5.94, p < .05).

The subjects in the touch group reported a stronger perception of the instructor's friendliness and helpfulness. A greater number of touch group respondents "agreed" concerning positive attitude toward the instructor than "disagreed" (χ^2 (1, N = 60) = 5.143, p < .05). Of those who agreed, significantly more of the touch group "strongly agreed" rather than "agreed" (χ^2 (1, N = 60) = 6.696, p < .01). (See Table 1 and Figure 1.)

The touch group subjects displayed more positive attitudes toward the task and were more motivated to work on the task for an extended period of time, with a difference between all four response categories (χ^2(3, N = 30) = 11.35 p < .01). More response variability characterized the touch group's reactions to a questionnaire

TABLE 1

CHI SQUARE

Perceptions of Instructor's
Friendliness and Helpfulness

	strongly agree	agree
touch	21	11
no-touch	9	19

χ^2(1, $\underline{N}$ = 60) = 6.696, $\underline{p}$ < .01

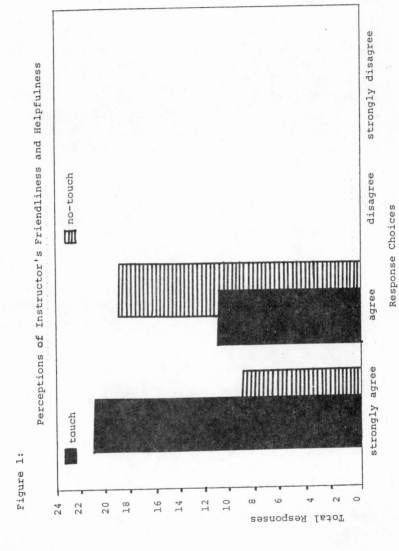

Figure 1:   Perceptions of Instructor's Friendliness and Helpfulness

item about their willingness to produce three more of the same product. (See Table 2 and Figure 2.)

Strong motivation to work with the instructor was found in the touch group. When asked to respond to the statement "I would love to work with this craft instructor every day," the touch group differed significantly from the no-touch group according to the "strongly agree" and "agree" response choices ($\chi^2(1, N = 27) = 5.040, p < .05$). (See Table 3 and Figure 3.)

Three statements regarding mood before, during, and after the craft session were analyzed. Although not statistically significant, 50% of the individuals in the touch group reported improved mood during or immediately after the craft session as compared to only 28.5% of the individuals who were not touched.

DISCUSSION

As reported in similar studies, significantly more touched subjects displayed positive attitudes toward the instructor and the task. Individuals agreed with descriptions of the instructor as both helpful and friendly. Similarly, subjects showed positive attitudes toward the task.

TABLE 2

CHI SQUARE

Attitudes toward the task

	strongly agree	agree	disagree	strongly disagree
touch	7	5	4	0
no-touch	0	3	9	2

$\chi^2(3, \underline{N} = 30) = 11.35, \underline{p} < .01$

Figure 2:

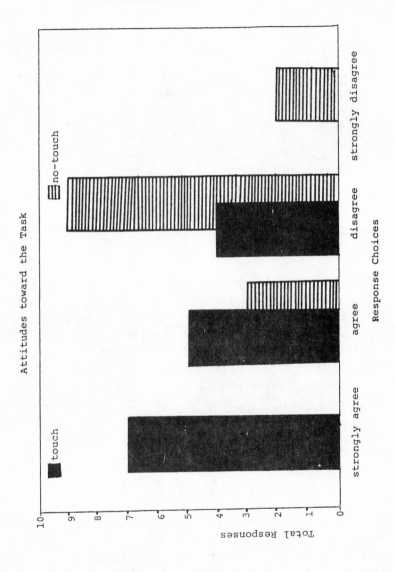

Attitudes toward the Task

43

TABLE 3

CHI SQUARE

Motivation to work for the Instructor

	strongly agree	agree
touch	8	6
no-touch	2	11

$\chi^2(1, \underline{N} = 27) = 5.040, \underline{p} < .05$

Touch was found to be a powerful influence on motivation for working with the instructor. When compared to no-touch respondents, a greater number of touch group respondents indicated they would want to work with the instructor every day. Subjects attending the craft session were able to receive unaccustomed, personal attention through the craft process. Receiving attention from a new instructor can have positive effects on individual responses toward motivation. Both the touch and no-touch groups received the same level of attention in the introduction of the project, but the touch group received additional attention through touch. Touching individuals can increase their desire to work for an occupational therapist.

Subjects in the touch group indicated greater motivation to work on a project for a specific period of time. However, results were ambiguous between the two groups regarding the self reported motivation to complete three more bookmark projects. Motivating a client to work on an activity seems to be easier if the project is completed and a different one started. Task duration was not a deterrent to the participant's continuing interest. Perhaps, it was the

Figure 3:   Motivation to work for the Instructor

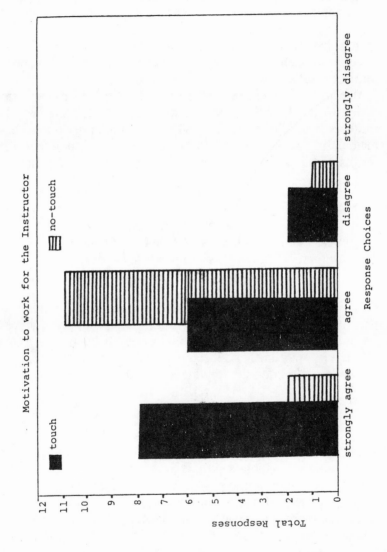

possibility of repeating equivalent projects within the same time period that the gerontic patients found to be less motivating.

Findings on mood indicate touch may play an important role in improving patients' moods while an activity is in progress. Research and development of a more sensitive measure of mood in relation to touch and, perhaps, the activity process might show significant results.

Due to the organization of the care facility, the participation of male patients would have incorporated extraneous variables into the study. Since Stein and Hall (1984) found similar responses between male and female subjects during touch studies, it is likely that the results of this study were not influenced by the exclusion of male subjects.

Suggestions for Further Research

Clinical evidence suggests that touch influences positive mood state. A more sensitive measure needs to be developed in order to find a direct relationship between the effects of touch and positive mood increases during an activity.

This study was implemented using a purposeful activity. The impact of touch on purposeful versus non-purposeful activity needs to be investigated. Research on the impact of touch regarding purposeful activity may further substantiate the occupational therapy profession's position on the importance of purposeful activity.

CONCLUSION

An occupational therapist's awareness and utilization of touch could increase a patient's attitude toward therapy and improve motivation. This study found that tactile stimulation positively impacts gerontic patient affect and motivation. Touch group respondents displayed a greater prevalence of strong, positive attitudes toward the instructor and the task as well as increased willingness to work for the instructor. The touched subjects showed greater motivation to work on a single task, or several different tasks, rather than many identical tasks within a specific amount of time. A touch on the shoulder is a positive influence on the gerontic person's attitude toward the task and therapist, and motivation to work for the instructor and complete an activity.

REFERENCES

Alagna, Frank J., Fisher, Jeffrey D., Whitcher, Sheryl J., & Wicas, Edward A. (1979). Evaluative Reaction to Touch in a Counseling Interview. *Journal of Counseling Psychology, 26*, 465-472.

Anderton, Charles H. & Heckel, Robert V. (1985). Touching Behaviors of Winners and Losers in Swimming Races. *Perceptual Motor Skills, 60*(1), 289-92.

Ayres, Jean A. (1979). *Sensory Integration and the Child*. Los Angeles: Western Psychological Services.

Burnside, I. M. (1973). Caring for the Aged: Touching is Talking. *American Journal of Nursing, 73*, 2060-63.

Cohen, Emory L., Lotyczewski, Bohdan S., & Weissberg, Roger P. (1982). Physical Contact in Interactions between Clinicians and Young Children. *Journal of Consulting and Clinical Psychology, 50*, 219-225.

Eyler, Steven C. (1983). Effects of Brief Touch during Individual Instruction. Unpublished Master's Thesis, University of Puget Sound, Tacoma, Washington.

Farber, Shereen D. (1982). *Neurorehabilitation a Multisensory Approach*. Philadelphia: W. B. Saunders Co.

Fisher, Jeffrey D. & Whitcher, Sheryl J. (1979). Multi-Dimension Reaction to Therapeutic Touch in a Hospital Setting. *Journal of Personality and Social Psychology, 37*, 87-91.

Fordyce, Jerry & Goldman, Morton (1983). Prosocial Behavior as Affected by Eye Contact, Touch, and Voice Expression. *Journal of Social Psychology, 121*, 125-129.

Frith, Greg H. & Lindsey, Jimmy D. (1983). Counselors, Handicapped Students, and the Touch Domain: A Recapitulation. *School Counselor, 31*, 34-9.

Heslin, Richard & Patterson, Miles L. (1982). *Nonverbal Behavior and Social Psychology*. New York: Plenum Press.

Huss, Joy (1977). Touch with Care or a Caring Touch? *American Journal of Occupational Therapy, 31*, 11-18.

Kleinke, Chris (1977). Compliance to Requests made by Gazing and Touching Experimenters in Field Settings. *Journal of Experimental Social Psychology, 13*, 218-223.

Montagu, Ashley (1978). *Touching*. New York: Harper and Row, Publishers.

Pattison, J. E. (1973). Effects of Touch on Self-Exploration and the Therapeutic Relationship. *Journal of Consulting and Clinical Psychology, 40*, 170-75.

Pertillo, Ruth (1978). *Health Professional/Patient Interaction*. Philadelphia: W. B. Saunders Co.

Preston, T. (1973). Caring for the Aged: When Words Fail. *American Journal of Nursing, 73,* 2064-66.

Rosenfield, Howard M. & Sussman, Nan M. (1978). Touch, Justification and Sex: Influences on the Aversiveness of Spacial Violations. *Journal of Social Psychology, 106,* 215-225.

Stein, D. S. & Hall J. A. (1984). Gender Differences in Touch: An Empirical and Theoretical Review. *Journal of Personality & Social Psychology, 47,* 440-459.

APPENDIX A

ATTITUDE QUESTIONNAIRE

Directions:
Circle the response you feel is most appropriate to the following statements.

1. I was in a great mood this morning.

   strongly agree   agree   disagree   strongly disagree

2. I felt the craft instructor was extremely helpful.

   strongly agree   agree   disagree   strongly disagree

3. I was in a bad mood during the craft session.

   strongly agree   agree   disagree   strongly disagree

4. I think the craft instructor was extremely friendly.

   strongly agree   agree   disagree   strongly disagree

5. I am in such a good mood right now, I feel like smiling the rest of the day.

   strongly agree   agree   disagree   strongly disagree

6. I wish I could work on this craft project for two more hours.

   strongly agree   agree   disagree   strongly disagree

7. I would love to work with this craft instructor every day.

   strongly agree   agree   disagree   strongly disagree

8. If this craft instructor asked me to make 3 more bookmarks I would gladly do so.

   strongly agree   agree   disagree   strongly disagree

APPENDIX B

Instructor's script

Good afternoon! My name is Debbie and I will be your craft instructor today. Before I begin with the instructions, I will tell you what we will be doing today. There are two parts to this project. During the first part, we will make a bookmark. I will give you instructions for the bookmark in a moment. During the second part you will fill out a questionnaire. When you are done or want to stop working on your bookmark, I would appreciate it if you would ask for and fill out a questionnaire. Are there any questions before I begin with the instructions to make the bookmark?

As I mentioned before, we are going to make a bookmark today. Here is a sample of a bookmark (instructor holds up sample for all to see). In front of each of you are materials to make a bookmark: pieces of felt, a felt pattern, scissors, and glue. You can either copy the sample by cutting out the pattern in front of you and glueing on pieces of felt provided, or make one of your own in order to complete the project. If you have any questions, do not hesitate to ask. Work at your own pace and use the materials provided to make your bookmark. I will walk around to see how everyone is doing. Are there any questions?

Thank you for joining us today!

A Group Psychotherapy Intervention to Promote the Functional Independence of Older Adults in a Long Term Rehabilitation Hospital: A Preliminary Study

Frima Christopher, PhD
Patricia Loeb, PhD
Herbert Zaretsky, PhD
Amir Jassani, MA

SUMMARY. As is true of the general population, older adults receive physical rehabilitation for deficits resulting from injury or disease. During the rehabilitation process, however, cognitive status and psychological well-being may be neglected and thus deteriorate during prolonged hospitalization. A group psychotherapy intervention utilizing insight and reminiscence was developed to offset the negative effects of institutionalization and to maintain or promote those qualities of survivorship (functional independence, self-determination and self-reliance) necessary for the geriatric patient's adjustment upon discharge to the community. Older adults were selected from those patients currently awaiting discharge from a rehabilitation hospital. All participants were pre- and post-tested by independent examiners with the Community Competence Scale. The findings suggest that this time-limited group intervention is important in the promotion of functional independence and further suggest that this approach can be modified to maximize the functioning of less competent, older adults.

The authors are affiliated with the Psychology Service, Department of Rehabilitation Medicine, New York University Medical Center, Goldwater Memorial Hospital, Roosevelt Island, NY 10044.

This is an adaptation of a paper presented at the 37th Annual Scientific Meeting of the Gerontological Society of America, San Antonio, TX, 1984.

Although institutionalization has provided an important rehabilitative environment for many older adults, problems secondary to long term placement may also surface and impact on patient improvement. Zaretsky and Brucker, 1976; Eisdorfer, 1977; and Lawton and Nahemow, 1973 have addressed the competing effects, positive and negative, of institutionalization. While long term placement provides the necessary intervention for multiple medical and psychosocial needs which emerge secondary to illness or injury (Grzesiak & Zaretsky, 1979) the patient is also vulnerable to further loss of adaptive functioning due to environmental factors (Lawton & Nahemow, 1973; & Lieberman, 1975) and age biases in the treatment process. Diagnoses of organically-based mental impairments, i.e., deficits of memory, orientation, or social adaptation (Perlick & Atkins, 1981) are assigned to institutionalized elderly persons more frequently than equally impaired community elderly (Sloane, 1980). As a result, discharge plans are modified or postponed. Extended hospitalization may further exacerbate those deficits in functioning which are the precursors of nonreversible deterioration (Eisdorfer, 1977; Lieberman, 1975; Libow, 1977) until discharge from long-term care no longer seems a viable option.

In order to maintain discharge as a feasible objective, institutions caring for the elderly must have as a focus the maintenance and development of the patients' competence and functional capacities. Institutional life, especially the psychological deprivation and dependency it often entails, may cause rapid deterioration of essential adaptive functioning and individual competence. In addition, maintenance of hospital routine and the tacit approval accorded compliant behaviors by staff may inadvertently foster dependence. Patient adjustment to the institutional routine may in fact be countertherapeutic. Skills and abilities necessary for life in the community are lost and consequent dependence on institutional care may result. It may be assumed, therefore, that where institutional programs are implemented to enhance competence and self-reliance, these detrimental effects may be reduced or eliminated. Specifically, the use of a group psychotherapeutic intervention has been determined to be an ecologically valid mechanism for intervention for this population (Yalom, 1983; Burnside, 1978). It provides a social microcosm of community interaction and permits a variety of insight/skills-based techniques to be incorporated within the context of the group (Christopher & Gugel, 1982).

The present study served as a preliminary investigation to explore the effectiveness of group psychotherapy in promoting the adaptive functioning of a select group of hospitalized older adults whose appropriateness for discharge was in question. Appropriateness for discharge was operationally defined as capacity for independent functioning, and was measured by the Community Competence Scale (CCS) (Loeb, 1983), an instrument useful in assessing functional competence. A time-limited psychotherapeutic group approach was devised, utilizing insight oriented interventions and structured as well as unstructured problem-solving strategies. It was believed that this approach would promote qualities of survivorship (functional independence, self-determination, and self-reliance) necessary for successful discharge.

METHOD

Subjects

Eight adults, aged 60 years and older, constituted the target group and were selected from a pool of 30 patients awaiting discharge. Each patient was screened to exclude individuals with a history of psychosis or developmental delay and any gross sensory impairments that would affect test administration and the ability to function in a group environment. These patients, four males (ages 73-82 years) and four females (age 56-77 years) had all sustained illness or injury requiring long term rehabilitation and each had been hospitalized for at least one year prior to the study's inception. The group was heterogeneous in terms of ethnicity, level of education, diagnosis/disability, and length of hospitalization (see Table I). All, with the exception of the college graduate, had held blue collar or small business positions.

Procedure

Thirty patients awaiting discharge were interviewed as potential participants in the group psychotherapy intervention. Twelve patients volunteered and agreed to participate in this investigation. Of

Table I

Demographic Charateristics of Group Participants

S	AGE	GENDER	EDUCATION	DIAGNOSIS/ DISABILITY	LENGTH OF HOSPITALIZATION
1	81	M	Elementary School	CA; prostate; renal edema metastic CA/Paraplegia	3 years
2	77	F	Elementary School	Right CVA; hypertension, ASHD/	3½ years
3	78	M	Sixth Grade	Right CVA, seizure disorder/ Left Hemiplegia	1½ years
4	73	M	10 yrs & Bus. School	Left BKA 2° to gangrene; partial amputation of right foot/ Bilateral hearing impairment	3 years
5	82	M	Eighth Grade	D.M., history of hypertension; S/P right BKA; TIA/	1 year
6	61	F	Some High School	S/P Left CVA with monoparesis; hypertension; S/P chronic renal failure/	2½ years
7	56	F	B.A.	Left CVA/Right hemiparesis, very mild aphasia	1½ years
8	62	F	Elementary School	S/P Left BKA 2° to gangrene, Hypothyroidism, D.M./	1½ years

these twelve, eight patients were available for the program's duration. Each participant was pre- and post-tested by graduate students in psychology trained in the administration and scoring of the Community Competence Scale (CCS) (Loeb, 1983). This instrument measures multiple dimensions of individual adaptive functioning. The CCS was selected because of its demonstrated value in assessing potential functional independence.

The CCS is comprised of 19 subscales (see Table II) which sample functional abilities in areas relevant to independent living. The 166 items of this test required the elderly person to actually demonstrate his or her abilities in each competence area. Responses were scored in relation to a standardized scoring system. Qualitative behavioral observations were also made and recorded in order to evaluate adaptive capabilities. A broad picture was thus provided of the older adult's information base, reasoning ability, and problem-solving capability in relation to many typical situations of daily life.

A time of eight weeks was established as best conforming to the

TABLE II

Subscales of the Community Competence Scale (Loeb, 1983)

Subscale Number	Name of Subscale
1.	Judgement
2.	Emergencies
3.	Acquire Money
4.	Compensate Incapacities
5.	Manage Money
6.	Communication
7.	Medical Care
8.	Memory
9.	Satisfactory Living
10.	Diet
11.	Mobility
12.	Sensation
13.	Motivation
14.	Hygiene
15.	Maintain Household
16.	Utilize Transportation
17.	Verbal/Math
18.	Social Adjustment
19.	Dangerousness

discharge calendar for these older adults. The group met twice weekly for a period of one hour and fifteen minutes with two senior staff psychologists as the group leaders. Each session encouraged interpersonal interaction, insight, and confrontation through a combination of leader-facilitated issue exploration and the fostering of a supportive climate. Problem identification, clarification of individual objectives and relevant coping strategies were also used to enhance adaptive functioning. More specifically, the content of the 16 sessions corresponded to the component areas of general competence reflected by the CCS subscales.

For example, several group sessions dealt with specific issues involving money management, while others focused on communication skills, and social adjustment. All the group sessions involved direct instruction, role playing and assigned homework, in addition to the exchange of interpersonal feedback. A detailed anecdotal record was maintained for the dual purpose of monitoring change over time and for tailoring the curriculum to the needs of the group members.

RESULTS

Although the statistical findings were not significant comparing total pre- and post-test scores on the CCS, several inferences may be drawn from the scores obtained from the competence measures. Five of the eight group participants scored at pre-test as dependent in functioning thus requiring the support services available in a Skilled Nursing Facility. Two participants reflected an inability to be self-monitoring. Support was required on an as-needed basis. One participant's score identified her as able to recognize problems and generate solutions, sustain objectives, and thereby demonstrate skills necessary for living independently within the community. At post-test, three patients improved in their CCS scores demonstrating an increased ability to function independently. One of these patients was subsequently discharged to the community. Improvement was most evident in subscales measuring more abstract areas such as attitudes and feelings of self-regard and less evident in areas measuring those concrete skills which rely on physical capacity as well as opportunity for continued use. Although the remaining five members post-tested shows gains in some areas of functioning, their overall scores showed little significant improvement.

Observational data, however, suggest areas of discernible patient improvement and little or no deterioration in psychological functioning. During the introductory phase of the group, members displayed a variety of egocentric behaviors including attentional deficits, parallel discursiveness, withdrawal, difficulty in focusing on interactional themes, resistance to establishing a group agenda, and a general unresponsiveness to establishing realistic limits. As the group evolved, and as the interpersonal dynamics became more open, issues involving competence and new learning became more easily integrated in the life course of the group. For example, the first session was characterized by defining personal objectives and combating the general: "I can't do it" attitude. For each patient, even simple tasks were viewed with extreme caution and skepticism. Using a hierarchical problem-solving model, the group segmented each task into more manageable domains of functioning. Thus, the breaking down of seemingly complex objectives into basic increments and establishing sequential opportunities for gain permitted patients of varying abilities to experience a renewed sense of competence. These included a range from the most basic: "How do I get my nurse to respect my possessions when they are in my drawer?" to the more complex: "If I want a book (on dogs), and I am immobilized in a hospital, how do I go about locating and ordering such a book?" The patient was encouraged to relearn telephone and budgeting skills. She independently confirmed the title, established the location of the text, determined price and thereupon negotiated the delivery and safe housing of this prized book. These skills are essential to life planning although observed gains may require alternative methods of measurement, e.g., checklists of in-group behaviors.

As the program evolved, there was a marked expansion of the group's initial focus. From the more concrete and manageable objectives, which dominated early sessions, emerged the more complex issue of discharge. Having been encouraged by tangible evidence of their own individual and collective competence, group members were better able to explore areas of independent functioning. Bolstered by increased self-esteem and situational clarity as well as by the group's support, the question of "how do I make a decision about when I am ready to go home (separate from and including medical considerations), and how do I choose where the next home is to be?" may be addressed. Thus, in areas where dependence on others was necessary, strategies were devised to maintain a balance between individual initiative and disability-specific needs. Increasingly, patients reported the ability to supplement their own efforts with appropriate requests for help from hospital personnel. Recognizing that their efforts to facilitate discharge could be enhanced, these patients were able to implement a campaign to help staff expedite the processing of their discharge plans.

Changes in member functioning were also observed outside the group. Records showed that as the group matured, individuals appeared better able to realistically appraise their own functioning in a variety of hospital settings. There were markers of increased involvement in hospital rehabilitation programs, and in decisions about personal health, although not all changes were in the direction of independent functioning. In one case, a patient experienced physical deterioration which offset cognitive and emotional gains. In another case, one patient deferred discharge in order to investigate alternatives to living alone in the community. Thus, a key finding was that group intervention provided a safe vehicle to explore a range of options, but that final decisions reflected individual personality, and did not always conform to expected measures of independence.

DISCUSSION

This study has attempted to explore the efficacy of a group therapy intervention in promoting functional independence for a group of elderly adults in long term chronic care. The results suggest that group psychotherapy is useful in maintaining or enhancing qualities of individual competence found to be likely to deteriorate upon prolonged institutionalization. The results further suggest that the changes in functioning observed within the group may generalize to the formulation of adaptive strategies outside the group. Even where physical disability and general psychological functioning served as barriers to maximum independent, members demonstrated an ability to achieve a more adaptive dependence. Thus, patients were better able to negotiate their needs within those constraints defined by their disability.

It is possible to infer from these findings that programs encouraging interpersonal interaction and the opportunity to exercise individual autonomy are useful in reconciling the competing demands of hospital regimen and personal objectives. On the other hand, the generalizability of an increase in individual autonomy may be limited by the incidence of psychological and/or medical deterioration as well as the institutional context in which behavior is expressed. The efficacy of any program whose goal it is to improve psychological functioning and promote functional adaptation must address the constraints imposed by changes in psychological and medical status and be integrated into a broad-based diagnostic and therapeutic milieu for positive change to be sustained over time. Otherwise, only short-term gains may be expected.

One problem in interpreting the findings of this investigation is that the observations are based on a relatively small subject sample, without a control group, using a short-term therapeutic intervention strategy. Thus, in order to generalize the observations to a wider population, additional research is needed. This research might include a broad-based diagnostic profile for each subject, the inclusion of more subjects, a post-treatment follow-up in order to measure the degree to which the effects are sustained over time (and in what conditions), the recording of in-group behavioral change, and the study of the relationship of other variables (affect, motivation, medical status, etc.) to the development of competence.

Another problem, one applicable to experimental research in general, concerns the utility of instruments selected to respond to the research questions. For example, the selection of an instrument designed to measure competence as if it were a uni-dimensional characteristic is complicated by the fact that competence, like any psychological variable, is essentially multi-faceted and complex. This issue, in part, explains the discrepancy that often arises between changes measured quantitatively and the perhaps more ecologically valid changes recorded via systematic observation. Even with observation, the relationship between noted changes and the efficacy of the treatment may be further complicated by the impact of variables not accounted for in the experimental design.

While these problems are important, the benefits of such an investigation as the present one are the findings which provide insight into issues central to the well-being of older adults in long term care. Interventions emphasizing the restoration of feelings of self-worth and independence have particular salience to this population because adaptive strategies developed over a lifetime may be lost as a result of prolonged hospitalization (Zaretsky & Brucker, 1976; Eisdorfer, 1977; Lawton & Nahemow, 1973). Institutions whose objective is recovery in its broadest definition will encourage the development of programs that further psychological well-being, such as group psychotherapy, in addition to the more traditional services designed to meet medical needs. This integrative approach, combining a gero-sensitive institutional policy, research, and treatment, may lead to improved standards for health service delivery for older adults.

REFERENCES

Bennett, R. and Eisdorfer, C. (1975). The institutional environment and behavior change. In S. Sherwood (Ed.), *Long-Term Care*. New York: Spectrum Publishing.

Burnside, I. M. (1978). Working with the elderly: Group process and techniques. North Scituate, Massachusetts: Duxbury Press.

Christopher, F. and Gugel, R. N. (1982). Therapeutic groups: A multidisciplinary, rehabilitative approach for the elderly. Paper/workshop presentation, Academy of Gerontological Education and Development, New York.

Eisdorfer, C. (1977). Stress, disease, and cognitive change in the aged. In C. Eisdorfer and R. O. Friedel (Eds.), *Cognitive and Emotional Disturbance in the Elderly: Clinical Issues*. Chicago, Illinois: Year Book Medical Publishers, Inc.

Grzesiak, R. C. and Zaretsky, H. H. (1979). Psychology in rehabilitation: Professional and clinical aspects. In R. Murray and J. C. Kijek (Eds.), *Current Perspectives in Rehabilitation Nursing*. St. Louis: The C. V. Mosby Co.

Lawton, M. P. and Nahemow, L. (1973). Ecology and the aging process. In C. Eisdorfer and M. P. Lawton (Eds.), *The Psychology of Adult Development and Aging*. American Psychological Association, Washington, D.C.

Libow, S. (1977). Senile dementia and "pseudosenility": Clinical Diagnosis. In C. Eisdorfer and R. O. Friedel (Eds.), *Cognitive and Emotional Disturbance in the Elderly: Clinical Issues.* Chicago, Illinois: Year Book Medical Publishers, Inc.

Lieberman, M. A. (1975). Adaptive processes in late life. In N. Datan and L. H. Ginsberg (Eds.), *Life-span Developmental Psychology: Normative Life Crises.* New York, Academic Press.

Loeb, P. A. (1983). Validity of the community competence scale with the elderly. Unpublished doctoral dissertation. St. Louis University.

Perlick, D. and Atkins, A. (1981). Variations in the reported age of patient: A source of bias in the diagnosis of depression and dementia. *Journal of Consulting and Clinical Psychology, 52,* 812-820.

Sloane, R. B. (1980). Organic brain syndrome. In J. E. Birren and R. B. Sloane (Eds.), *Handbook of Mental Health and Aging.* Englewood Cliffs, New Jersey: Prentice Hall.

Yalom, I. D. (1983). In-patient group psychotherapy. New York: Basic Books, Inc.

Zaretsky, H. H. and Brucker, B. S. (1976). Verbal discrimination learning as a function of brain damage, aging, and institutionalization. *The Journal of General Psychology, 95,* 303-312.

The Effectiveness
of an Occupational Therapy Program
in an Inpatient Geropsychiatric Setting

Rosalie S. Lushbough, MS, OTR
J. Michael Priddy, PhD
Hobart H. Sewell, MD
Stephen B. Lovett, PhD
Theresa C. Jones, OTR

SUMMARY. Twelve patients in an inpatient geropsychiatric facility participated in a specially designed program of occupational therapy and psychosocial groups. A matched set of twelve patients participated in the regular treatment program of the facility, but not in the special program. All subjects were rated on the Comprehensive Occupational Therapy Evaluation, the Nurses Observation Scale for Inpatient Evaluation, and the Brief Psychiatric Rating Scale before and after the four-month program. Participants in the special program showed significant improvement on ratings of interpersonal effectiveness, and clinically demonstrated increased responsibility for the group attendance and appropriateness in group participation. No significant differences were noted on overall ratings of psychiatric dysfunction. Implications of the study for group leaders and for further research are discussed.

The effectiveness of occupational therapy and psychosocial interventions with geropsychiatric populations is an area of promise that deserves systematic exploration. In general, the literature in this area is limited, and lacks both good experimental design and clear outcome measures (Gilewski, 1986). However, there are clinical indications that a variety of psychosocial interventions are effective in alleviating symptoms and improving functional level in the geropsychiatric population.

Mental health disciplines use various approaches in the treatment of geropsychiatric patients. Each field has its own body of literature that supports its particular interventions and theoretical bases. The occupational therapy literature focuses on the effectiveness of activity versus verbal groups, while the psychotherapy literature investigates different psychotherapeutic techniques for relative effectiveness. DeCarlo and Mann (1985) found that activity therapy was significantly more effective than verbal therapy in improving self-perceptions of interpersonal communication skills with psychiatric patients in a day treatment center. In this setting, activities provided opportunities for the participants to work through many of their difficulties with interpersonal communication. Klyczek and Mann (1986) compared outcome measures from a day treatment center offering primarily an activity-oriented approach with a center offering a verbally-oriented approach. Activities included: traditional crafts, parties, dinners, games, sports, and cultural/educational trips. Verbal therapies included insight-oriented discussions and paper-and-pencil tasks. Comparison of the group means showed that clients receiving activity therapy achieved a four times greater symptom reduction. This translates to increase independent functioning in the areas of self-esteem, decision making, leisure time use, and occupational or life role adjustment.

An investigation of the effectiveness of a new social activities program in a nursing home revealed that over a six-month period, patients who participated in the study demonstrated improved moods and decreased feelings of loneliness (Arnetz, 1985). The activity level of the treatment group increased threefold over the same period of time, and patients maintained their internal locus of control.

Most of the occupational therapy approaches utilize movement and media which draw upon sensory and cognitive resources. For the very cognitively impaired geriatric patient, sensory stimulation has been found to be useful in forestalling deterioration, rekindling an interest in the environment, and bringing about specific behavioral improvements. Paire and Karney (1984) developed a sensory stimulation program in which group members were presented with olfactory, visual, auditory, tactile, kinesthetic, and gustatory stimulus items and then discussed their associations with these stimuli. Results measured by the Geriatric Rating Scale indicated that within twelve weeks, patients in the sensory stimulation group improved in daily hygiene skills and showed renewed interest in group and social affairs.

The positive results of these studies indicate a need for more information on which types of therapy work best with which populations, about which settings. Gugel (1986) reviewed the following therapeutic intervention approaches for data on effectiveness: reality orientation, stimulation programs, behavior therapy, and psychotherapy. The data on reality orientation groups are equivocal and do not indicate that significant gains in orientation can be made using this technique. Stimulation programs, including body movement and perceptual and cognitive activities, have generally used subjective evaluations and the therapeutic effect of the intervention is unclear. The behavior therapy approach focuses on changing non-functional behavior to functional behavior. This approach appears to be most effective in the social, self-care, and purposeful areas of behavior, and least effective in changing cognitive and emotional functioning. Psychotherapy includes a range of techniques, from active interviews to confrontation and reality testing. Group psychotherapy is the most common format for institutions. Typical results are improved overall behavior, cognitive function, sociability, self-concept, discharge rates, and decreased depression (Parham, Priddy, McGovern, & Richman, 1982). In a study of the treatability of 96 mentally impaired, institutionalized elderly, Gugel (1979) found that an insight-oriented group psychotherapy approach resulted in significant increases in social involvement and self-esteem, responsibility for self, independence in ADLs, improved physical mobility, and increased discharge rates.

Gilewski (1986) reviewed the literature on group therapy with cognitively impaired older adults covering the last 35 years. He found that most of the groups studied used a variety of techniques to arrive at specific goals. The most frequently reported benefits of psychosocial intervention were improved patient and staff morale and improved cognitive and behavioral functioning for patients. According to Gilewski, nothing conclusive can be found regarding the effectiveness of group therapy with cognitively impaired older adults, although the trends that were reported included some success with each group, and no negative results have been reported.

Levy, Derogatis, Gallagher, and Gatz (1980) pointed out that no long-term benefit has been observed in behavioral and psychotherapeutic interventions with the cognitively impaired elderly, and that therapy with this population serves to reduce symptoms and optimize present functioning rather than to produce improvements and cures.

In contrast, Feil (1983) found that change in behavior with the disoriented elderly was slow, but that a six-month validation group led to less incontinence, improved speech, less crying, and more talking and helping others. Significant affective changes were also reported. Using validation therapy techniques in groups, Feil found that by acknowledging group members' feelings, she could help them to diminish feelings of anxiety and concomitant disorientation. She noticed that when patients felt validated and nurtured, they became able to think more logically, even leaving their disoriented world and returning to present reality. Her approach to group work included music, movement, topic discussions, and refreshments.

PROGRAM DESIGN

Patients in the geropsychiatric population usually operate with the cognitive liability of being unable to plan beyond their immediate situation or to remember directions for use at a later time (Levy, 1986). Essential activities must be structured and scheduled for them. Certain activities can be selected to maintain present skills and to promote a sense of competence and success in the midst of confusion. These may include sports, arts and crafts, writing, dancing, music, cooking, and cleaning. Besides requiring success-oriented activities, patients need to have their feelings validated and their individual problems addressed. with this characteristic to consider, a program was designed to meet the activity and psychosocial needs of an inpatient geropsychiatric population and to measure the effects of the intervention.

SETTING

The present study was conducted at Bay HealthCare (BHC), a 50 bed, for-profit locked geropsychiatric facility in Palo Alto, California. As is the case with most small, private psychiatric facilities, the population represents a spectrum of late-life disorders. These include residual schizophrenia, bipolar disorders, major depression, late life paranoia, and a variety of organically based impairments, such as Alzheimer's Disease and alcohol-related dementia. The median age at BHC is 68; men and women are equally represented. As a facility with the designated goal of geropsychiatric rehabilitation, the optimum length of stay is considered to be six to nine months. In reality, some BHC patients are ready to return to a less restrictive living environment in two or three months, while others have remained in the facility for several years.

The program staff at BHC is responsible for all therapeutic activities, and consists of a psychiatrist, a psychologist, two occupational therapists, an activities director, and volunteers. A structured program of activities is provided seven days a week. Each patient receives individualized activity and behavior management treatment plans, which are reviewed and updated at least once every three months. While individual and family therapy are available, the primary treatment modalities are group and milieu interventions; groups are designed to meet the various needs of different subsets of the population, with discussion and community living skills training for the more cognitively intact patients and movement and sensory stimulation for the more severely impaired.

Psychotropic medications are used conservatively at BHC. The philosophy of the treatment team is that it is preferable to cope with mild agitation or disordered thinking than to risk a further compromise of cognitive functioning through overmedication. In addition, many BHC patients have long histories of institutionalization and phenothiazine use, and the risk of tardive dyskinesia is significant.

THE INTERVENTION

The fundamental hypothesis of this study was that a specifically designed set of occupational therapy and psychosocial groups would result in improved functioning for the higher functioning BHC patient. Accordingly, a five-group package was structured as follows:

— Stress Management. Facilitated by the staff psychologist, this intervention focused on stressful events within the hospital, and assisted patients in the development of more effective strategies (e.g., assertion, relaxation) to cope with these stressors.
— Arts and crafts. Staff occupational therapists worked with patients on individualized craft projects to promote personal expression and to increase self-esteem.
— Sports. All staff joined patients in outdoor physical activity, such as "nerf" football and volleyball.
— Creative Pen. In this group, patients were given specific writing assignments designed to stimulate creative thinking. Some topics were based on reminiscence, while others were devoted to the expression of fantasy.
— Goals group. In Goals group, patients set personal goals, either within the facility or for community living. Impediments to reaching these goals were discussed, the necessary intermediate steps identified, and strategies formulated for reaching the goal.

Finally, patients were offered opportunities to have "one-to-ones." All participants in the study were encouraged to have frequent brief individual sessions ("one-to-ones") with the research staff. These sessions focused on topics of the patient's choosing, and were frequently combined with shopping trips or other community outings.

The non-study participants also participated in "one-to-ones" and were encouraged to attend groups led by the activities director and the nurses aides, including outdoor walks, music socials, bingo, current events, and money management.

POPULATION

Twelve patients were selected by Lushbough and Priddy as meeting the minimum criterion set: the capacity to achieve maximum benefit from the predesigned treatment package. This group consisted of eight men and four women, average age 61 years. Most were diagnosed as having functional psychiatic disorders, as opposed to more organic impairment; several, however, had dual diagnoses.

As selection of the treatment group was not random, matched controls were selected from the remaining BHC population. The matched group was selected on the bases of age, length of hospitalization, diagnosis, and general functional level. As stated, the treatment group was composed of twelve patients who were felt to be best suited for the study; as a result, a difference on pretest measures was expected, and incorporated into the design and data analysis.

METHODOLOGY

The special group series was conducted for a four-month period. Prior to the initiation of the groups, pretest data were collected on the twelve study patients and the twelve matched controls. The measures used included the Comprehensive Occupational Therapy Evaluation (COTE) (Brayman & Kirby, 1983), the Brief Psychiatric Rating Scale (BPRS) (Overall, 1962), and the Nurses Observation Scale for Inpatient Evaluation (NOSIE) (Honingfeld & Klett, 1965). On all three of these measures, lower scores indicate psychosocial improvement. The COTE scale consists of 25 behavioral items in subcategories of general, interpersonal, and task behaviors. The BPRS consists of 18 items in the categories of anxiety and depression, anergia, thought disturbance, activation, hostility and suspiciousness. The NOSIE contains 32 items in the areas of social competence, social interest, personal neatness, cooperation, irritability, manifest psychosis, and depression. The BPRS and NOSIE scales were completed by the staff psychiatrist and director of nurses, respectively; both were blind to the assignment of patients to treatment and control conditions. All patients were reassessed at the conclusion of the program with the same measures. Clinical data were also collected on the patients, including medications received by each patient at the initiation and conclusion of the study.

During the study period, group leaders completed an attendance sheet at the conclusion of each session; study patients attending groups were rated on a three-point scale for level of participation and appropriateness.

RESULTS

T-test scores for the treatment and control groups from the pre-intervention assessment demonstrated no significant differences between groups at the beginning of the intervention.

Separate Analysis of Covariance (ANCOVA) tests were conducted for each key assessment variable to determine if the groups differed in extent of psychopathology at post-intervention when pre-intervention levels of pathology were controlled. Pre-intervention scores were used as covariates. The results indicated that treatment subjects obtained lower post-intervention scores on the COTE interpersonal subscale than did controls. T-tests between pre- and post-intervention scores for each group on this subscale revealed that the treatment subjects demonstrated a significant decrease in scores while the control group remained unchanged. The decrease in scores on the interpersonal subscale indicates significant improvement. No other measures demonstrated significant treatment effects.

It was hypothesized that the subjects' level of attendance and appropriate participation in the treatment programs would be positively associated with improvement in their degree of psychopathology. Three variables were created to test this hypothesis: the total number of treatment sessions attended; the mean rating of amount of participation at each session; and the mean rating of appropriateness of participation at each session. These three ratings were correlated with pre- to post-intervention changes in the outcome measures for the twelve treatment subjects. The results indicated that subjects who attended the most treatment sessions demonstrated the greatest reduction in psychopathology on the NOSIE mental health rating (i = − .62, p < (.03)).

DISCUSSION

Results of the data analysis reveal an improvement in interpersonal relations, a skill directly relevant to the nature of the interventions. Differential improvement, however, did not generalize to more global ratings of independence, functional level, and self care as measured by the NOSIE, nor to overall level of psychiatric impairment as measured by the BPRS. Clinically, there was observable improvement in several areas, including voluntary group attendance, patient-to-patient interactions in groups, and sustained task-oriented behavior. Perhaps most significantly, two of the treatment group patients were successfully placed in less restrictive levels of care during the time of the study, as opposed to none of the controls. Nevertheless, the fact remains that there were no significant changes on two of the three outcome measures used.

There are several possible explanations for the lack of significant change on the NOSIE and the BPRS. Both scales have been used in a wide variety of psychiatric settings. The population of BHC, however, represents a particularly chronic subsection of psychiatric patients, with symptomatology perhaps too severe to be affected by a short-term intervention to a degree reflected in a global measure of functioning. In addition, both scales, to be sufficiently sensitive to the changes observed, may require more extensive rater training than was possible within the confines of the present study. Instruments specifically targeted to the proposed goals of the intervention may also be more appropriate than the more general functional ratings of the NOSIE and the BPRS.

The significant change on the COTE interpersonal scale is encouraging. The chronic mental patient, after years of institutionalization, as a rule has minimal social skills. Apathy and passivity characterize the interpersonal style of most BHC patients. It has been gratifying to observe an increase in relevant interpersonal behavior among patients, both in and out of groups. Interpersonal skills are also directly related to readiness to function in a less restrictive level of care. Passivity may be adaptive on a chronic mental ward, but a more active level of interpersonal involvement is essential to functioning in the community. Improvement in this area alone would seem to make the package of group interventions used in the current study a successful endeavor.

Several recommendations for further research follow from the current study. As mentioned, specific rather that global outcome measures should be used whenever possible, and multiple and carefully trained and monitored raters should be employed. A larger, more carefully controlled study might be able to determine which components of the current intervention package were most directly related to the positive changes noted. Finally, studies drawing research populations from a larger universe of subjects might be able to formulate more homogeneous treatment groups, decreasing within-group variance caused by a multiplicity of diagnoses. In essence, the current research is best viewed as an applied pilot study, generating promising initial data to be explored further in a more formal research setting.

CONCLUSIONS

A package of psychosocial and occupational therapy interventions was applied to a small group of institutionalized psychogeriatric patients. These patients, after four months in the special treatment program, demonstrated improved interpersonal skills and appeared clinically to be functioning at a higher overall level than a group of matched controls. Global psychiatric and nursing skills, however, failed to indicate significant change. The current research project raises interesting possibilities for more extensive and carefully controlled research.

REFERENCES

Arnetz, B.B. (1985). Gerontic occupational therapy: Psychological and social predictors of participation and therapeutic benefits. *American Journal of Occupational Therapy, 39,* 460-465.

Brayman, T., and Kirby, J. (1983). The comprehensive occupational therapy evaluation. In B. Hemphill, (Ed.), *The evaluative process in psychiatric occupational therapy.* New York: Slack.

DeCarlo, J.J., and Mann, W.C. (1985). The effectiveness of verbal versus activity group in improving self-perceptions of interpersonal communication skills. *American Journal of Occupational Therapy*, *39*, 20-27.

Feil, N. (1983). Group work with disoriented nursing home residents. In S. Shura (Ed.), *Groupwork with the frail elderly*. New York: Haworth.

Gilewski, M.J. (1986). Group therapy with cognitively impaired adults. In T.L. Brink (Ed.), *Clinical gerontology: A guide to assessment and intervention*. New York: Haworth.

Gilewski, M.J. (1986). Group therapy with cognitively impaired adults. In T. L. Brink (Ed.), *Clinical gerontology: A guide to assessment and intervention*. New York: Haworth.

Gugel, R.N. (1979). The effects of group psychotherapy on orientation, memory, reasoning ability, social involvement, and depression of brain damaged and non-brain damaged aged patients exhibiting senile behavior. *Dissertation Abstracts International*, *90*, 172.

Gugel, R.N., and Eisdorfer, S.E. (1986). Psychological interventions. *Topics in Geriatric Rehabilitation*, *1*, 27-34.

Honingfeld, G., and Klett, C.J. (1965). The nurses observation scale for inpatient evaluation. *Journal of Clinical Psychology*, 21, 65-71.

Klyczek, J.P., and Mann, W.C. (1986). Therapeutic modality comparisons in day treatment. *American Journal of Occupational Therapy*, 40, 606-611.

Levy, L.L. (1986). A practical guide to the care of the Alzheimer's Disease victim: The cognitive disability perspective. *Topics in Geriatric Rehabilitation*, *1*, 16-22.

Levy, S.M., Derogatis, L.R., Gallagher, D., and Gatz, M. (1980). Intervention with older adults and the evaluation of outcome. In L.W. Poon (Ed.), *Aging in the 1980s: Psychological issues*. Washington, DC: American Psychological Association.

Overall, J.F., and Gorham, D.R. (1962). The brief psychiatric rating scale. *Psychiatric Reports*, *10*, 799-812.

Paire, J.A., and Karney, R.J. (1984). The effectiveness of sensory stimulation for geropsychiatric inpatients. *American Journal of Occupational Therapy*, *38*, 505-509.

Parham, I.A., Priddy, J.M., McGovern, T.V., and Richman, C.M. (1982). Group psychotherapy with the elderly: Problems and prospects. *Psychotherapy: Theory, Research and Practice*, *19*, 437-443.

ANOTHER PERSPECTIVE

"A Thousand Small Deliberations"*

Sherry Hoff

Oh, why was he here?
He hadn't planned to live this long.
When had he gotten old?*

He was 92 years old and upset. He shouldn't be in the hospital. He wasn't really sick, nothing that going home couldn't cure. How could all these young hospital people know what HE needed? How could they presume to imply that it might not be "safe" for him to return to his own home? Hadn't he been on his own since he was 14, even learning to cook after his wife died three years ago? Hadn't he faced and solved more problems than anyone would ever know? This time should be no different.

He had just taken a little step the wrong way, not looking where he was going. That could happen to anyone. He had fallen before but this time he had gotten caught, his hip was broken. He had been in the hospital long enough, if they would just send him home he knew he could mend even faster and never let it happen again. To top it off though, they had said he would have to quit driving. He had been driving years, before all these hospital people were born.

---

*T. S. Eliot, "Gerontion"

He had a perfect record too. So he had missed a couple curbs lately, he really only needed to drive to the grocery store. He never drove very fast or very far.

How could he be old, already?

He, the sturdy child who was born and raised in a sod hut on the Midwestern plains. The hut that would keep out the rains of spring but not the rattlesnakes of summer. And in winter would allow the blowing snow to sift into his room at night and dust his bed.

This same child that spent those many wonderful Christmases at his cousin's. The journey there would take all day, thirty miles in the family buckboard. The night before, his mother would heat great tubs of grain to take along. While they traveled they would all take turns dipping their icy feet into the warm tingling kernels.

The young man who came West to Oregon to work in the great timber forests. He had come to be a pretty good spar tree topper, climbing to the tip of the biggest and strongest trees and sawing off the top by hand. When the top let loose it took a mighty strong man to hang on while the trunk snapped and whipped in recoil from the insult.

Then war. Time to fight for his country.

France in 1917. There is very little to be said. There was too much loss. In those days the only medical treatments available for a wounded soldier were iodine, epsom salts, and castor oil. He had been lucky.

Then the good years, before the Depression. He had met and married his wonderful wife. She could bake bread like nobody else. They had never bought a loaf of bread. Until, of course, she had become ill. They had two children, one gone already, the other still young but sickly.

The thirties. Many a better man than he had failed to provide for his family during those hard times. The Depression was tougher on the Easterners and the Southerners than those out West. The Westerners had land and room to spread out. They could hunt, fish, farm, and even raise a few head of cattle. A man could always trade crops and get by. He had had a fair sized orchard. There were no apple buyers, but rather than throw the fruit out he had given it away or traded for the few staples they needed to get by.

Time went by too quickly after that. Already it had been 25 years since he had retired. What had they done in those years? They had traveled. They had taken that big car trip the year after he retired. His wife had been from Oregon and always wanted to see the country. Later he had been quite content working in his wood shop out back. Making tables, clocks, birdhouses and what-nots had been very rewarding until his hands had gotten too shaky and things didn't turn out the way he wanted.

Then his wife had gotten sick. He took care of her until she died. She had been a talented lady, an artist. She taught art to the women of their small community. People loved her and her work. He was lonely and still missed her.

After she had died he didn't go out quite as much. It wasn't so hard to get by. Without her some of the old chores really didn't need doing and he could still do what he wanted. He liked to just sit and read the *Readers Digest* or watch a little TV. In the summer he had planted big gardens. That might be hard to do this year but maybe a few tomatoes.

Then he had fallen again. He didn't even know how it happened. He had laid there for many hours. He didn't hurt but he couldn't move. The phone was out of reach. His neighbor had come for his regular visit and found him.

That was months ago. Things weren't moving as swiftly as he'd planned. In fact they weren't moving at all in the hospital. His doctor told him the hip wasn't healed well enough for him to walk on, just yet. Then he had gotten that bad cold. Sure he was weak and just dressing was a chore but he was better now, getting stronger every day. Surely strong enough to go home. He knew everything would work itself out if only he could go home. His had been a lifetime of hard times and hard work. Things had been tough before but he had been tougher. He would show them, he would be tough again. He was patient and not afraid of hard work. He would go home someday.